PCEP

Perinatal Continuing Education Program

Specialized Newborn Care

BOOK III

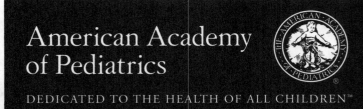

American Academy of Pediatrics

DEDICATED TO THE HEALTH OF ALL CHILDREN™

PCEP

The original version of these self-instructional books was developed in 1978 at the University of Virginia under contract (#N09-HR-2926) from the National Heart, Lung, and Blood Institute. Subsequent versions have been developed independently by the authors.

John Kattwinkel, MD
Lynn J. Cook, RNC, MPH
Hallam Hurt, MD
George A. Nowacek, PhD
Jerry G. Short, PhD

Primary authors for the obstetrical content

Warren M. Crosby, MD
Lynn J. Cook, RNC, MPH

The neonatal resuscitation information in these books is written to be consistent with the national guidelines approved by the following groups:
American Academy of Pediatrics
American Heart Association
American College of Obstetricians and Gynecologists

Several different approaches to specific perinatal problems may be acceptable. The PCEP books have been written to present specific recommendations rather than to include all currently acceptable options. The recommendations in these books should not be considered the only accepted standard of care. We encourage development of local standards in consultation with your regional perinatal center staff.

Library of Congress Control Number: 2006929345

ISBN-13: 978-1-58110-218-5
ISBN-10: 1-58110-218-6

PC0004

Copyright © 2007 by the University of Virginia Patent Foundation.

All rights reserved.

Permission is granted to reproduce individual tables and charts in limited quantities for use within a health care facility. This book, units within the book, and skill units may not be reproduced.

The PCEP books are one part of a larger perinatal program. Information about the books, and the educational program, may be obtained by visiting the PCEP Web site at www.pcep.org.

Brand names are furnished for identification purposes only. No endorsement of the manufacturers or products is implied.

1 2 3 4 5 6 7 8 9 10

Continuing Education Credit

Continuing education credit is available for every perinatal health care provider who studies the Perinatal Continuing Education Program (PCEP) books. These American Medical Association (AMA) credits or contact hours/continuing education units (CEUs) are available to physicians, nurses, nurse practitioners, certified nurse midwives, respiratory therapists, and any other professional who provides care to pregnant women or newborn babies.

American Medical Association

Accreditation Statement

The University of Virginia School of Medicine is accredited by the Accreditation Council for Continuing Medical Education (ACCME) to provide continuing medical education for physicians.

The University of Virginia School of Medicine designates this educational activity for a maximum of 51 *AMA PRA Category 1 Credit(s)™*. Physicians should only claim credit commensurate with the extent of their participation in the activity.

The University of Virginia School of Medicine awards 0.1 CEU per contact hour to each nonphysician participant who successfully completes this educational activity. The CEU is a nationally recognized unit of measure for continuing education and training activities that meet specific educational planning requirements. The University of Virginia School of Medicine maintains a permanent record of participants who have been awarded CEUs.

Conflict of Interest Disclosures

As a provider accredited by the ACCME, the Office of Continuing Medical Education of the University of Virginia School of Medicine must ensure balance, independence, objectivity, and scientific rigor in all its individually sponsored or jointly sponsored educational activities. All faculty participating in a sponsored activity are expected to disclose to the activity audience any significant financial interest or other relationship (1) with the manufacturer(s) of any commercial product(s) and/or provider(s) of commercial services discussed in an educational presentation and (2) with any commercial supporters of the activity (significant financial interest or other relationship can include such things as grants or research support, employee, consultant, major stock holder, member of speakers bureau, etc). The intent of this disclosure is not to prevent a speaker with a significant financial or other relationship from making a presentation, but rather to provide listeners with information on which they can make their own judgments. It remains for the audience to determine whether the speaker's interests or relationships may influence the presentation with regard to exposition or conclusion.

The University of Virginia School of Medicine, as an ACCME provider, requires that all faculty presenters identify and disclose any off-label uses for pharmaceutical and medical device products. The University of Virginia School of Medicine recommends that each physician fully review all the available data on new products or procedures prior to instituting them with patients.

John Kattwinkel, MD, has disclosed no significant financial relationships with manufacturers of products discussed in these materials and has disclosed no off-label uses of any US Food and Drug Administration (FDA)-approved pharmaceutical products or medical devices.

Lynn J. Cook, RNC, MPH, has disclosed no significant financial relationships with manufacturers of products discussed in these materials and has disclosed no off-label uses of any FDA-approved pharmaceutical products or medical devices.

Hallam Hurt, MD, has disclosed no significant financial relationships with manufacturers of products discussed in these materials and has disclosed no off-label uses of any FDA-approved pharmaceutical products or medical devices.

George A. Nowacek, PhD, has disclosed no significant financial relationships with manufacturers of products discussed in these materials and has disclosed no off-label uses of any FDA-approved pharmaceutical products or medical devices.

Jerry G. Short, PhD, has disclosed no significant financial relationships with manufacturers of products discussed in these materials and has disclosed no off-label uses of any FDA-approved pharmaceutical products or medical devices.

Warren M. Crosby, MD, has disclosed no significant financial relationships with manufacturers of products discussed in these materials and has disclosed no off-label uses of any FDA-approved pharmaceutical products or medical devices.

AMA PRA Category 1 Credit(s)™ or Contact Hour Credit

Credit is given only for complete books, not individual educational units. Possible hours: Book I, 10.5; Book II: Maternal and Fetal Care, 15.0; Book II: Neonatal Care, 15.0; Book III, 10.5.

Required submission items

1. *Pretest and posttest answer pages* for *EACH* book studied (at the end of each book)

2. *Evaluation form* (precedes answer pages at the end of each book)

3. *Continuing education credit registration form* (ONE form per submission) (download from www.pcep.org/cec.html)

4. *Payment,* according to information given on the continuing education credit registration form (www.pcep.org/cec.html) is required.

PCEP

Perinatal Continuing Education Program

BOOK I

Maternal and Fetal Evaluation and Immediate Newborn Care

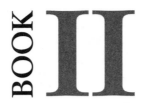

Maternal and Fetal Care

BOOK II

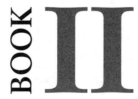

Neonatal Care

BOOK II

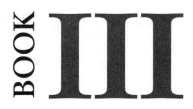

BOOK III

Specialized Newborn Care

Unit 1

Review: Is the Baby Sick? Identifying and Caring for Sick and At-Risk Infants

Objectives

In this unit you will

A. *Review the concepts* taught in Book I: Is the Mother Sick? Is the Fetus Sick? and Is the Baby Sick?

B. Review the situations in which **anticipation** of problems is most important.

C. Review the situations in which **immediate action** is most important.

D. Learn how to **decide what to do first** when a sick baby has more than one problem.

E. Work through a **realistic clinical case example** to apply the information learned in the previous units to the care of newborns in your hospital.

Unit 1 Pretest

Before reading the unit, please answer the following questions. Select the *one best* answer to each question (unless otherwise instructed). Record your answers on the answer sheet that is the last page in this book *and* on the test.

1A. A 4,000-g (8 lb, 13 oz) baby girl is born in your hospital to a woman who was diagnosed with abnormal glucose tolerance at 24 weeks' gestation. She had a cesarean delivery at 36 weeks because of abnormal stress test results. The Apgar scores were 8 at 1 minute and 9 at 5 minutes. The baby is pink and active, with the following vital signs: pulse = 140 beats per minute, respirations 40 = breaths per minute and unlabored, temperature = 36.5°C (97.7°F), blood pressure 46/36 mm Hg. What should be done for this baby?

Yes No
___ ___ Place the baby in supplemental oxygen.
___ ___ Do a gestational age and size examination.
___ ___ Obtain a blood glucose screening test.
___ ___ Start an intravenous line and give 8 mL of 10% glucose.
___ ___ Repeat vital signs frequently.

1B. It is quite likely that this baby is

Yes No
___ ___ Small for gestational age
___ ___ Preterm
___ ___ Large for gestational age
___ ___ Post-term

1C. The baby is at risk for developing the following:

Yes No
___ ___ Hypoglycemia
___ ___ Diarrhea
___ ___ Meconium aspiration
___ ___ Respiratory distress syndrome
___ ___ Neonatal diabetes mellitus

1D. At 4 hours of age the baby's vital signs are normal, and she continues to look well. By this time, assuming no further information is available, the following should have been done already or would now be appropriate to do.

Yes No
___ ___ Start oral feedings (breast or bottle).
___ ___ Begin antibiotic therapy.
___ ___ Place under phototherapy lights.
___ ___ Repeat blood glucose screening test.
___ ___ Give oxygen.
___ ___ Treat like a healthy baby.

2A. An 1,800-g (4 lb) 3-day-old, 33-week estimated gestational age baby has been in your care in the nursery. She has been feeding well, has had no respiratory problems, and is appropriate size for gestational age. Because of her size and gestational age, she has been continuously connected to a cardiorespiratory monitor. Between feedings, she suddenly becomes apneic, cyanotic, and limp, with a heart rate of 50 beats per minute. She does not resume breathing with vigorous stimulation. For each item, mark the line in the *one* most appropriate column.

Do Immediately	Do in Next Several Minutes	Not Indicated	
_____	_____	_____	Obtain blood glucose screening test.
_____	_____	_____	Give epinephrine 0.5 mL (1:10,000).
_____	_____	_____	Connect an oximeter to the baby.
_____	_____	_____	Assist ventilation with bag and mask.
_____	_____	_____	Stimulate with warm water.
_____	_____	_____	Obtain a hematocrit.
_____	_____	_____	Check blood pressure.
_____	_____	_____	Obtain a blood gas.
_____	_____	_____	Take the baby's temperature.

2B. What are the possible reasons for this baby's difficulties?

Yes	No	
___	___	Common problem of prematurity
___	___	Sepsis
___	___	Hypoglycemia
___	___	Aspirated formula
___	___	Blood oxygen too high

For each question, please make sure you have marked your answer on the test and on the answer sheet (last page in book). The test is for you; the answer sheet will need to be turned in for continuing education credit.

This unit is an expansion of the concepts you learned in Book I. It is also a review of many of the ideas you learned in previous units.

To determine if a baby is sick, at risk, or well, do 2 things.

- Review the baby's history.
- Examine the baby.

1. How Do You Know an Infant Is Well?

A. History

Consider all of the risk factors that you have learned for each of the perinatal periods.
- Maternal history
- Labor and delivery history
- Neonatal history

B. Physical Examination

A well baby
- Is 38 to 42 weeks' gestational age at birth
- Is an appropriate size for gestational age
- Has normal
  - Heart rate
  - Respirations
  - Temperature
  - Blood pressure
  - Color
  - Activity
  - Feeding pattern
- Passes meconium within the first 24 hours
- Urinates within the first 24 hours

 A well baby has no risk factor in any of the perinatal periods; is term and appropriate for gestational age (AGA); has normal vital signs, color, activity, and feeding; and has normal stool and urine output.

2. How Do You Know an Infant Is At Risk?

An at-risk baby is one who has a greater chance of developing problems, either because of risk factors in the baby's history and/or because of the baby's size or gestational age. An at-risk baby's well-being depends on

- Continued careful assessment
- Anticipation of problems that are likely to occur
- Prevention of these problems or immediate treatment of them, should they occur

An at-risk infant needs continued monitoring for potential problems, but does not need immediate treatment for any problem.

A. History

    1. Abnormal Prenatal and/or Neonatal History

    Consider all of the risk factors for each of the perinatal periods.

      • Maternal history

      • Labor and delivery history

      • Neonatal history

    2. Previously Sick Baby

    Babies who were sick but now have normal vital signs, color, activity, and feeding pattern are also at-risk babies.

B. Physical Examination

    An at-risk baby

    • Is preterm or post-term

    and/or

    • Large for gestational age (LGA) or small for gestational age (SGA)

    • Has normal

      – Heart rate

      – Respirations

      – Temperature

      – Blood pressure

      – Color

      – Activity

      – Feeding pattern

    • Passes meconium within the first 24 hours

    • Urinates within the first 24 hours

 An at-risk baby has normal vital signs, color, activity, and feeding, with normal stool and urine output, but is preterm or post-term; and/or SGA or LGA; and/or has prenatal or neonatal risk factors; and/or is a baby recovering from having been sick.

3. How Do You Know an Infant Is Sick?

A. History

    A sick baby may be

    • A well baby, without any identified risk factors, who suddenly develops abnormal vital signs, color, activity, or feeding pattern

    • An at-risk baby whose condition deteriorates

    or

    • A baby sick from birth

B. Physical Examination

The items to consider in your initial examination include

Heart Rate:
- Tachycardia (>180 beats per minute [bpm])
- Bradycardia (<100 bpm)
- Persistent murmur

Respirations:
- Tachypnea (sustained respiratory rate >60 breaths/minute)
- Gasping
- Apnea
- Grunting, retracting, or nasal flaring

Temperature:
- High
- Low
- Unstable

Blood Pressure:
- Hypotension
- Poor capillary refill time
- Weak pulses

Color:
- Cyanotic
- Pale, gray, or mottled
- Red
- Jaundiced

Activity:
- Tremors, irritability, seizures
- Floppy, decreased muscle tone
- Little response to stimulation

Feeding:
- Poor feeding
- Abdominal distention
- Recurrent vomiting

 A sick infant has abnormal vital signs, color, activity, and/or feeding pattern and needs immediate action from you to stabilize the baby, investigate the cause, and treat the abnormality.

Self-Test

Now answer these questions to test yourself on the information in the last section.

A1. It is useful to think of 3 "types" of babies because they require different types of care. List 3 types.

_____

_____

_____

A2. Well babies are term and appropriate for gestational age. List 3 other characteristics of well babies.

_____

_____

_____

A3. At-risk babies have normal vital signs. List 4 other characteristics at-risk babies may have.

_____

_____

_____

_____

A4. List 6 characteristics sick babies may have.

_____

_____

_____

_____

_____

_____

Check your answers with the list near the end of the unit. Correct any incorrect answers and review the appropriate section in the unit.

4. What Should You Do for a Well Baby?

A well baby may become sick. For this reason, you should *routinely assess* the condition of all well babies by checking their temperatures, heart rates, and respiratory rates at least once every 8 hours. Well babies may receive breastfeedings or bottle-feedings using a normal routine. Color, activity, and feeding pattern should be carefully assessed. If a well baby does become sick, this will be evident by changes in vital sign(s), color, activity, or feeding pattern of the baby.

5. What Should You Do for an At-Risk Baby?

The key to management of an at-risk baby is to *anticipate problems* so that they may be avoided or corrected quickly. To do this, you should perform certain tests frequently to *monitor risk factors*. For example, an LGA baby is at risk for hypoglycemia. You would anticipate this and obtain blood glucose screening tests.

6. What Should You Do for a Sick Baby?

Once you have determined that a baby has abnormal vital signs, color, activity, or feeding pattern, and therefore have classified the baby as sick, you must *act quickly* to correct these abnormalities.

You need to do 3 things for sick babies.

1. *Treat the immediate problem.*

2. *Determine why* the baby is sick and *treat the cause* when it is found.

3. *Monitor risk factors* so that potential problems can be prevented or treated promptly.

For example

- An LGA baby suddenly turns blue and has a seizure. You immediately give oxygen until the baby is pink. *(Treat immediate problem.)*

- You then obtain a blood glucose screening test and vital signs. You attach a cardiorespiratory monitor to the baby. You find that the blood glucose screening test result is 0 to 20 mg%. *(Determine why the baby is sick.)*

- You quickly send a blood sample for blood glucose determination, insert a peripheral intravenous (IV) line or umbilical venous catheter, give 10% glucose (2 mL/kg), and then begin a constant infusion of 10% glucose. *(Treat the cause of the abnormality.)*

- Twenty minutes later, you obtain another blood glucose screening test and find that it is 80 to 120 mg%. You continue to obtain blood glucose screening tests every 30 to 60 minutes for several hours, then at longer intervals. *(Monitor risk factor.)*

7. How Do You Decide What to Treat First?

The care of sick babies may seem extremely complicated. At times it may seem difficult to decide what action to take first when an infant with multiple risk factors suddenly becomes apneic or cyanotic or has a seizure. Remember, no matter what the cause of the problems, the first thing you should *always* do is check the baby's *Airway, Breathing, and Circulation, then Stabilize* the baby.

Remember these ABCS

A. *Airway:*   Make sure there is no obstruction to airflow into the baby's lungs.

B. *Breathing:*   Give oxygen by oxyhood or assist the baby's breathing with bag and mask, or endotracheal tube and bag breathing, as necessary.

C. *Circulation:* Check the baby's heart rate and blood pressure. If abnormal, take immediate action to correct them.

Then

S. *Stabilize:*

    1. Check: • All vital signs

                  • Hematocrit

                  • Blood glucose screening test

    2. Restore them to normal or as near normal as possible.

    3. Connect a cardiorespiratory monitor to the baby, and usually a pulse oximeter too.

    4. Decide exactly what other problems or risk factors the baby has and begin evaluation and treatment of those.

8. What Should You *Avoid* Doing When Caring for At-Risk and Sick Babies?

You have learned many actions you should take to care for at-risk and sick babies. Certain actions, however, may make these babies worse. Below is a list of "*Don'ts.*"

A. Feeding

Sick babies should *not* be fed either by nipple or tube feedings until their vital signs are stable. In general, sick babies should have IV feedings started early and continued for several days. A sick baby may aspirate if fed by mouth. Later, after their vital signs have stabilized, they may be given tube feedings.

B. Bathing

Sick and at-risk babies should *not* be bathed until their vital signs have been stable for several hours; even then a bath is not a necessary part of the baby's care. The vernix (material covering the baby's skin before birth) may help to prevent infection and does not need to be washed off quickly after birth. Baths should be delayed until the baby is completely stable because a bath can be stressful and easily cause a baby to become hypothermic.

C. Administering Oxygen

Sick babies do *not always* require oxygen. Oxygen given to sick babies who have normal lungs has been associated with eye damage (retinopathy of prematurity). Always determine the need for oxygen before giving it. If a baby needs oxygen, however, it should be given immediately.

D. Removing Oxygen

Sick babies who require oxygen should *not* be removed from oxygen for x-rays, weighing, or *any reason.* Any baby who requires oxygen may become much worse if taken out of oxygen for even a few moments.

E. Gestational Aging and Physical Examination

Sick babies should *not* have a detailed physical and neurologic examination until their vital signs are stable. Sick babies require gentle care; any excessive stimulation may cause them to become sicker. When the baby is stable, a gentle examination may be done.

F. Handwashing

Sick and preterm babies are more susceptible to infections. By far the most common way infections are transmitted among babies and from staff members to babies is lack of careful handwashing and/or lack of consistent use of a waterless antiseptic agent.

Do *not forget* to wash your hands or use a waterless antiseptic agent before and after each time you examine or care for each baby. Cleansing of hands and standard precautions are needed at all times, for all babies, by all providers.

9. How Do You Determine Why a Baby Is Sick?

You need to assess the baby's

- *Risk factors:* You should learn the risk factors (if any) for every baby delivered in your hospital. This includes reviewing each baby's prenatal, labor and delivery, and neonatal histories.

- *Vital signs and observations:* Temperature, pulse, respirations, and blood pressure should be taken at least once an hour for every sick baby. At-risk babies also require frequent checking of vital signs. Color and activity should be assessed carefully and routinely.

- *Laboratory tests:* The appropriate tests depend on a baby's risk factors and/or illness. Proper care of an at-risk or sick baby requires that appropriate tests be done, even if a baby "looks OK."

Self-Test

Now answer these questions to test yourself on the information in the last section.

B1. What are the ABCS that help you decide what to do first when caring for sick babies?

A. _____

B. _____

C. _____

S. _____

B2. What are 6 things you should *not* do for sick babies?

_____

_____

_____

_____

_____

_____

B3. What are the 3 main tools you use to assess a sick baby?

_____

_____

_____

Check your answers with the list near the end of the unit. Correct any incorrect answers and review the appropriate section in the unit.

Subsection: Vital Signs and Observations

Review the *observe*, *think*, and *act* categories for each vital sign, as well as color, activity, and feeding. **Some material in this and the subsequent section appears nowhere else in the Perinatal Continuing Education Program books.**

Heart Rate (Normal is approximately 120–160 bpm.)*

Observe	Think	Act
Tachycardia (>180 bpm)	• Hypovolemia • Anemia • Acidosis • Sepsis • Hyperthermia • Congestive heart failure • Arrhythmia	• Attach oximeter. • Check hematocrit, blood pressure, blood gas, temperature. • Consider cultures and antibiotics. • Electrocardiogram if rate >220.
Bradycardia (<100 bpm)	• Hypoxia • Hypothermia[†] • Acidosis • Sepsis • Congenital heart block	• Attach oximeter. • Give oxygen, as indicated. • Check arterial blood gas, temperature. • Consider cultures and antibiotics. • Electrocardiogram if persistent.

Murmurs	• Functional
	• Congenital heart disease
		• If murmur persists, obtain chest x-ray and echocardiogram, if available.
		• If baby cyanotic
		  – Give oxygen and check arterial blood gas.
		  – Consult cardiology or regional center staff.

*Newborn heart rates and respiratory rates are variable and should be counted for *1 full minute*. Assess the whole baby when interpreting a high or low heart or respiratory rate.
[†]Warm a severely chilled infant according to guidelines in Book II: Neonatal Care, Thermal Environment.

Temperature (Normal is approximately 37°C [98.6°F].)

Observe	Think	Act
Hyperthermia (>37.5°C = 99.6°F)	• Overheated environment • Sepsis (rarely)	• Check environmental temperature. • Consider cultures and antibiotics.
Hypothermia (<36.5°C = 97.7°F) or Unstable temperature	• Sepsis • Shock • Acidosis • Excessive heat loss • Necrotizing enterocolitis	• Check environmental temperature. • Check and correct routes of heat loss. • Check blood pressure, blood gas, white blood cell (WBC) count with differential. • Warm baby.* • Consider cultures and antibiotics. • Consider abdominal x-ray.

*Warm a severely chilled infant according to guidelines in Book II: Neonatal Care, Thermal Environment.

Blood Pressure (Normal varies by gestational age and postnatal age.)*

Observe	Think	Act
Below normal range	• Shock from blood loss • Sepsis • Acidosis • Poor oxygenation • Poor cardiac output	• Check arterial blood gas, hematocrit, WBC count with differential. • Attach oximeter. • Give volume expander (10 mL/kg) slowly, if indicated (suspected hypovolemia). • If blood loss suspected, send blood sample for type and crossmatch. • Consider cultures and antibiotics. • Administer oxygen as indicated.

*Refer to graphs in Book II: Neonatal Care, Blood Pressure.

Respirations (Normal is approximately 20–60 breaths per minute.)*

Observe	Think	Act
Grunting, flaring, retractions, or tachypnea (sustained respiratory rate >60)	• Respiratory distress syndrome • Transient tachypnea • Meconium aspiration • Pneumonia • Pneumothorax • Airway obstruction • Sepsis • Shock • Hypoglycemia • Polycythemia • Anemia • Hypothermia • Hyperthermia • Diaphragmatic hernia • Tracheoesophageal fistula • Congenital heart disease	• Attach oximeter. • Give oxygen as indicated. • Check blood pressure, arterial blood gas, blood glucose screening test, hematocrit, chest x-ray, temperature, WBC count with differential. • Roughly estimate gestational age and size. • Review history. • Consider cultures and antibiotics. • Consider assisted ventilation.
Gasping	• Severe acidosis	• Attach oximeter. • Obtain blood gas, especially check pH. • Consider assisted ventilation.
Apnea	• Worsening respiratory distress • Low blood oxygen • Hypoglycemia • Sepsis • Other significant illness (eg, necrotizing enterocolitis) • Shock • Acidosis • Low calcium • Low sodium • Central nervous system disorder • Cold-stressed baby rewarmed too rapidly† • Preterm	• Attach oximeter. • Consider assisted ventilation. • Check blood pressure, temperature, blood glucose screening test, hematocrit, arterial blood gas, chest x-ray, calcium, sodium, WBC count with differential. • Consider lumbar puncture. • Obtain cultures and start antibiotics. • Review history.
Severe respiratory distress at birth	• Choanal atresia	• Attempt to pass nasogastric tube. If nasogastric tube will not pass, place oral airway.
	• Diaphragmatic hernia	• Sunken abdomen: intubate and bag-breathe, insert nasogastric tube, position baby in 45° head-up angle, obtain chest x-ray.
	• Robin anomaly	• Place baby prone; consider placing large-bore (12F) nasopharyngeal tube.

*Newborn heart rates and respiratory rates are variable, and should be counted for *1 full minute*. Assess the whole baby when interpreting a high or low heart or respiratory rate.

†Warm a severely chilled infant according to guidelines in Book II: Neonatal Care, Thermal Environment.

Color

Observe	Think	Act
Cyanotic	• Respiratory distress • Hypoxia • Hypoglycemia • Acidosis • Hypothermia • Sepsis • Heart disease • Pneumothorax (especially with sudden cyanosis)	• Give oxygen. • Attach oximeter. • Ventilate as indicated. • Check temperature, arterial blood gas, hematocrit, blood glucose screening test, chest x-ray, echocardiogram (if available), WBC count with differential. • Consider cultures and antibiotics.
Pale, pallor	• Shock • Anemia • Sepsis	• Attach oximeter. • Check blood pressure, hematocrit, arterial blood gas, WBC count with differential. • Give volume expander and/or packed red blood cells as indicated. • Consider cultures and antibiotics.
Red	• Polycythemia • Overheated baby • Severe hypothermia	• Check hematocrit. • Check baby's temperature and environmental temperature.
Yellow (jaundiced)	• Liver immaturity or injury • Hemolysis • Sepsis	• Check vital signs, bilirubin, smear of peripheral blood, Coombs tests, reticulocytes, mother's and baby's blood type. • Consider cultures and antibiotics. • Assess baby's hydration. • Assess feeding pattern. • Investigate signs of congenital infections. • Assess medication history in baby.
Mottled, gray	• Acidosis • Hypotension • Hypothermia • Sepsis	• Attach oximeter. • Check arterial blood gas, blood pressure, temperature, WBC count with differential. • Consider cultures and antibiotics.

Activity

Observe	Think	Act
Decreased muscle tone or decreased reflex irritability, lethargy	• Sepsis • Hypoglycemia • Acidosis • Shock • Birth trauma • Central nervous system hemorrhage • Intrapartum maternal medications	• Consider cultures and antibiotics. • Consider lumbar puncture. • Check blood pressure, WBC count with differential, blood gas, blood glucose screening test, hematocrit. • Review maternal medications during labor. • Consider cranial ultrasound.

Increased activity (tremors, irritability, seizures*)	• Hypoglycemia
	• Low serum calcium
	• Meningitis
	• Complications of perinatal compromise
	• Drug withdrawal
		• Check blood glucose screening test, serum calcium.
		• Consider lumbar puncture.
		  – *High WBC count*: Culture spinal fluid and treat the baby with antibiotics.
		  – *Bloody*: Suspect birth trauma.
		• Assess maternal drug history.
		• Consider toxicology screen of baby's urine.

*Treat definite seizures *immediately*. Give phenobarbital 20 mg/kg, intravenously. Be prepared to ventilate if respiratory depression occurs. Provide maintenance dose of 3.5 to 5 mg/kg/day. Check serum levels and readjust dose as necessary to maintain serum level of 15 to 40 mcg/mL.

Feeding

Observe	Think	Act
Poor	• Sepsis • Complications of perinatal compromise	• Check temperature, hematocrit, arterial blood gas, blood pressure, blood glucose screening test. • Consider cultures and antibiotics. • Start IV.
Recurrent vomiting, abdominal distension	• Sepsis • Gastrointestinal obstruction • Necrotizing enterocolitis	• Check temperature, blood pressure, hematocrit, arterial or venous blood gas (check pH, especially), blood pressure, blood glucose screening test, WBC count with differential. • Consider cultures and antibiotics. • Pass nasogastric tube ($\geq$8F) and connect to low constant suction. • Obtain chest and abdominal x-ray. • Withhold feedings. • Start IV.
Excessive mucus and/or difficulty feeding	• Tracheoesophageal fistula	• Insert nasogastric tube ($\geq$8F), connect to low constant suction. • Obtain x-ray, look for nasogastric tube coiled in blind pouch. • Do *not* give barium or dye. • Withhold feedings, start IV. • Position baby at 45° head-up angle.
Recurrent, excessive residual amount (found in stomach before tube feeding)	• Necrotizing enterocolitis • Sepsis • Ileus	• Check temperature, hematocrit, arterial blood gas, blood glucose screening test, WBC count with differential. • Consider cultures and antibiotics. • Consider abdominal x-ray and nasogastric tube drainage.

Subsection: Tests and Results

The tests that follow are blood, cerebral spinal fluid, and urine tests, then abdominal and chest x-rays. *Only those tests with values and corresponding actions that can be put concisely in chart form are given.* For other blood tests and how to interpret and respond to results, such as bilirubin, see Book II: Neonatal Care.

 Some tests, and guidelines for response to results, are given only here, not in any previous units.

A. Blood Gas Values (See also Book II: Neonatal Care, Oxygen and Respiratory Distress.)

Blood gases measure the oxygen, carbon dioxide, and pH of blood. An arterial blood gas (ABG) is needed to measure blood oxygen. However, a venous or capillary blood gas provides a fair estimate of carbon dioxide, pH, and bicarbonate.

For an acutely ill baby, obtain an ABG measurement every 4 hours, and 10 to 30 minutes after each significant change in the baby's environmental oxygen concentration. If a pulse oximeter is used, more or less frequent ABG determinations may be needed, depending on the stability of oxygenation and the need to evaluate pH and carbon dioxide levels.

Acceptable Blood Gas Values

	Arterial		Capillary		Venous
PaO_2	45–75 mm Hg	PaO_2	Unreliable	PaO_2	Unreliable
pH	7.25–7.35	pH:	7.25–7.35	pH	7.25–7.35
$PaCO_2$	40–50 mm Hg	$PaCO_2$	40–50 mm Hg	$PaCO_2$	40–50 mm Hg
HCO_3^-	19–22 mm Hg	HCO_3^-	19–22 mm Hg	HCO_3^-	19–22 mm Hg

Note: The values shown are general guidelines only. There is controversy about what values constitute normality and what maximum and minimum values should be tolerated under various circumstances and conditions.

Blood Gas Test Results and Recommended Responses

Test	Abnormal Blood Gas Result	Action
PaO_2	• >75 mm Hg (high)	• Lower oxygen concentration until PaO_2 is 45–75 mm Hg.
	• <45 mm Hg (low)	• Give sufficient oxygen to bring PaO_2 to 45–75 mm Hg.
$PaCO_2$	• >55 mm Hg (high)	• Obtain arterial blood gas measurements frequently. • Consider intubation and assisted ventilation if $PaCO_2$ continues to rise and pH is <7.25.
	• <35 mm Hg (low)	• Look for reason for hyperventilation. • Consider possibility of metabolic acidosis or low PaO_2.
pH	• <7.25 (low)	• If (1) baby's ventilation is adequate and (2) bicarbonate level is <15–16 mEq/L, consider giving sodium bicarbonate while determining and treating cause of the acidosis. • If $PaCO_2$ is >60 mm Hg, consider assisted ventilation.
HCO_3^- (Bicarbonate)	• <16 mEq/L (low)	• If $PaCO_2$ is normal or low, consider administering sodium bicarbonate while determining and treating cause of metabolic acidosis. • If $PaCO_2$ is >60 mm Hg, do not administer sodium bicarbonate. Treat the high $PaCO_2$ with assisted ventilation and recheck blood gases.

B. Oxyhemoglobin Saturation and PaO_2.*

Oxyhemoglobin Saturation   *PaO_2*

Low = 0%–85% ------------------- 0–45 mm Hg

Desirable range = 85%–95% ------------------- 45–75 mm Hg

High = 95%–100% ------------------ 75–600 mm Hg

Figure 1.1 shows an approximation of the curve that could be constructed from the results of blood drawn from a slightly preterm

---

*The precise relationship of oxygen saturation and PaO_2 is affected by several factors such as gestational age, age since birth, and whether the baby has had a blood transfusion.

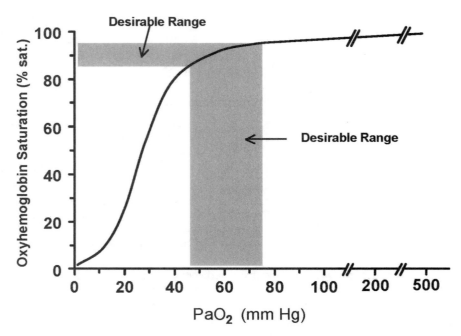

Figure 1.1. Oxyhemoglobin Dissociation Curve

baby during the first few days after birth. For some babies, simultaneous measurements of PaO_2 and oxygen saturation may give results quite different than those predicted by the graph.

Oxyhemoglobin saturation as measured by a pulse oximeter is most valuable for detecting *low* blood oxygen. It is *not* a sensitive measure for *high* blood oxygen, and provides no information about pH, carbon dioxide, and serum bicarbonate levels.

C. Blood Glucose Screening Test

Blood Glucose Screening Test (Normal value is 45–130 mg%.)

Screening Test Results	Actions
<20–25 mg%	1. Draw blood glucose. 2. Start IV with 10% glucose. Give 2 mL/kg over 5 minutes. 3. Run IV at 5 mL/kg/hour 4. Obtain another screening test or blood glucose level within 15–30 minutes. If test result remains <20–25 mg%, 15% glucose may be needed. 5. Begin frequent feedings as soon as blood glucose is normal, baby is stable, and baby is able to feed. 6. Monitor with frequent blood glucose screening tests.

Between 20–45 mg%	1. Draw blood glucose.
	2. Begin early, frequent feedings (immediately or at least within 4 hours of birth).
	3. Supplement with IV of 10% glucose if
	  • Feedings not tolerated
	  or
	  • Blood glucose remains 20–45 mg%
	4. Monitor with frequent blood glucose screening tests.

Between 45–90 mg%	1. Begin early, frequent feedings (within 4 hours of birth)

D. Electrolytes

Electrolytes are usually checked in any baby who experienced perinatal compromise, had seizures, has a gastrointestinal problem, or who requires IV fluids for more than 24 hours. There may be other abnormalities of electrolytes as a result of complex disease processes. These abnormalities are not discussed here.

Normal Values*

Sodium	133–148 mEq/L
Potassium	4.5–6.6 mEq/L
Chloride	100–115 mEq/L
Bicarbonate	19–22 mEq/L
Calcium (total)	8.0–11.0 mg/100 mL
Calcium (ionized)	4.0–4.7 mg/100 mL

Electrolytes

Abnormal Result*	Action
Low sodium	Decide if the baby has received too much IV fluid in the face of a poor urinary output. Decide if the baby has not received enough sodium, or is losing sodium (eg, stool, ileostomy).
High sodium	Suspect that the infant may have gotten too much sodium in the form of IV fluids or sodium bicarbonate. Stop excess sodium being administered. Suspect the baby (especially a very preterm baby) may be dehydrated and consider increasing fluid intake.
Low bicarbonate	See Blood Gas Test Results earlier in this section
Low calcium	Low calcium levels are not uncommon in preterm babies or in babies who required prolonged resuscitation and received sodium bicarbonate. In general, if the total serum calcium is <7 mg/100 mL or ionized calcium is <3.5 mg/100 mL and there are any symptoms of hypocalcemia (seizures or jitteriness), treatment is recommended. You should give 200 mg/kg of calcium gluconate, *slowly,* intravenously as a starting dose or 500 mg/kg/day intravenously as a maintenance dose.
	When calcium is given intravenously, you must *monitor the baby's heart rate*. If the heart rate begins to decrease during the infusion, **stop the infusion**. You should also make *certain the IV is not infiltrated* because calcium may cause severe tissue damage.

*Normal values may vary laboratory to laboratory. Check the ones used by your laboratory.

E. Hematocrit: Normal value is 45% to 65% (first day after birth).

The hematocrit or hemoglobin of a baby's blood tells you if the baby has anemia or polycythemia. Depending on results, you may want to give blood, or even take blood away.

When evaluating for polycythemia, **obtain hematocrit samples only from a vein**. A sample obtained from a heel stick may be extremely inaccurate during the first several days of life.

Hematocrit

Abnormal Result	Action
High: >65%–70%	*Polycythemia:* May lead to sludging of blood in the capillary beds of the lungs and brain. If the baby has symptoms and/or the high value has been confirmed by a repeat determination, a type of exchange transfusion can be done to lower the hematocrit by removing some to the baby's blood and replacing it with normal saline (also called a reduction or dilutional exchange transfusion). See Unit 4, Exchange, Reduction, and Direct Transfusions.
Low: <30%–35%	*Anemia:* Type and crossmatch the baby's blood and consider giving packed red blood cells (10 mL/kg) if baby is <2 days of age and in distress (increased heart rate, respiratory distress), or if the hematocrit is falling rapidly.

F. Platelet Count: Normal value is 150,000 to 450,000/μL.

Characteristically in newborns, the platelet count will fall acutely in response to a variety of illnesses, and then may become abnormally high as the baby recovers. The baby's platelets may also be low because of certain maternal drugs; specific maternal conditions, such as pregnancy-specific hypertension; or an antibody that the mother may have made against the baby's platelets.

Platelet Count

Abnormal Result	Action
<150,000/μL	*Thrombocytopenia:* Decreasing platelets can be an indicator of illness such as infection. Administration of platelets is usually not necessary, however, unless the count becomes extremely low or the baby shows signs of bleeding. • Look for signs of infection and consider obtaining other tests for infection. • Review maternal history for low platelet count, preeclampsia, bacterial or viral infection or other illness, or drugs associated with low platelets. • Recheck the platelet count. Monitor baby and obtain further studies depending on results and baby's clinical condition.
<100,000/μL	If there are signs of bleeding (eg, petechiae, gastrointestinal blood, oozing needle puncture sites, etc), consider administering platelets. Consult with your regional center about appropriate diagnostic studies that should be obtained prior to a platelet transfusion.
<25,000/μL	Platelets below 100,000/μL are abnormal at any gestational age. Many experts advise administering platelets if the count in below 25,000/μL, even if there is no evidence of bleeding. Consult with regional center staff about appropriate diagnostic studies that should be obtained prior to a platelet transfusion.

G. Spinal Fluid Tests

The spinal fluid is obtained from a lumbar puncture, usually obtained because infection (meningitis) is suspected. Several tests may be performed on the fluid. White blood cells, red blood cells, and bacteria can be identified with a microscope. Spinal fluid glucose and protein can be measured. If you suspect infection, spinal fluid should be cultured.

Normal Values (during first day after birth)

White blood cells	0–26
Red blood cells	0–600
Glucose	38–64 mg%
Protein	40–140 mg%

Spinal Fluid Tests

Abnormal Result	Action
Increased white cells	Think of infection. Culture and treat with antibiotics.
Red blood cells	Think of birth trauma, central nervous system hemorrhage, or a traumatic lumbar puncture.
Bacteria	Think of infection. Culture and treat with antibiotics.
Low glucose	Think of low blood glucose or infection. Culture and treat with antibiotics. Obtain blood glucose screening test and manage according to results.
High protein	Think of birth trauma, a central nervous system hemorrhage, or infection.

H. Urine Tests

Urine may be examined under a microscope to determine if there are red blood cells, white blood cells, or bacteria in the urine. When infection is suspected, a urine sample obtained by bladder catheter or suprapubic tap should be cultured.

Urine Tests

Abnormal Result	Action
White blood cells	Think of infection. Obtain cultures. Consider beginning antibiotics.
Red blood cells	Think of severe perinatal compromise. Consider restricting fluids.
Bacteria	Think of infection. Consider obtaining blood and urine cultures, and beginning antibiotics.

I. X-rays

Chest X-rays

Chest x-rays help you decide the cause of respiratory distress and determine the severity of the problem.

Abdominal X-rays

Abdominal x-rays help you decide the cause of vomiting, "spitting," abdominal distension, or a sunken abdomen. If an umbilical catheter is in place, it will be visible on the x-ray and should be checked for proper positioning.

Chest X-rays

Abnormal Result	Action
Respiratory distress syndrome	Treat as indicated in Book II: Neonatal Care, Respiratory Distress. Cannot be distinguished from bacterial pneumonia and sepsis. Consider cultures and antibiotics.
Transient tachypnea of the newborn	Treat respiratory distress as indicated in Book II: Neonatal Care, Respiratory Distress.
Pneumothorax	A small pneumothorax may not need treatment if blood gases are normal and baby is in no distress. Otherwise, insert needle and aspirate air if the baby is in distress and a chest tube is not immediately available; when available, insert chest tube and connect to underwater seal and appropriate suction apparatus.
Pneumonia	Obtain cultures. Treat with antibiotics.
Meconium aspiration	Treat respiratory distress as indicated in Book II: Neonatal Care, Respiratory Distress. Consider cultures and antibiotics.
Diaphragmatic hernia	Insert 8F (or larger) nasogastric tube and aspirate air from stomach. Leave tube in place, unclamped or connected to suction. Position baby at 45° head-up position. Do not use bag-and-mask assisted ventilation. Intubate if baby is in respiratory distress. Consult regional center staff immediately regarding surgery and possible transport of the baby to an extracorporeal membrane oxygenation (ECMO) center.
Tracheoesophageal fistula	Insert nasogastric tube. Aspirate air and fluid frequently or connect to suction. Position baby in 45° head-up position. Do not feed, do not give barium or dye. Consult a pediatric surgeon immediately.
Abnormal heart configuration	Obtain • Arterial blood gas • Blood pressure in arms and legs (4 extremities) • Echocardiogram • Pre- and post-ductal pulse oximetry (right hand and 1 leg)

Abdominal X-rays

Abnormal Result	Action
Intestinal obstruction	Stop feedings. Insert nasogastric tube and connect to suction. Consult pediatric surgeon immediately.
Necrotizing enterocolitis (dilated loops of bowel with air in intestinal wall)	Make NPO. Insert nasogastric tube and connect to suction. Obtain cultures and begin antibiotics. Monitor vital signs. Record intake and output. Consult regional center.
Umbilical arterial catheter too high or too low	Adjust or replace catheter so that catheter tip lies between the 3rd and 4th lumbar vertebrae.
Umbilical venous catheter too high or too low	Adjust or replace catheter so that catheter tip lies in the inferior vena cava.

Figure 1.2 is an expansion of the one presented in Book I, Is the Baby Sick? It summarizes the recommended approach to all newborn babies.

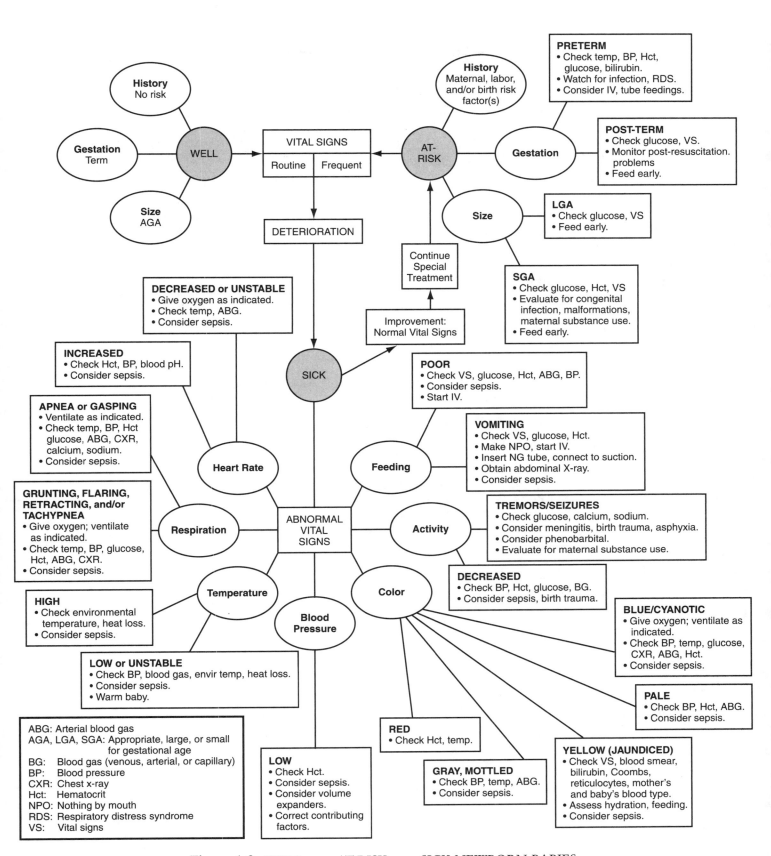

Figure 1.2. WELL ⟷ AT-RISK ⟷ SICK NEWBORN BABIES

Sample Case

This case sample will give you practice testing your knowledge, as well as provide experience in considering multiple factors that go into the care of at-risk and sick women and newborns. ***You should use the material within this unit to help you answer the questions.***

A woman pregnant with her fourth child is admitted to your hospital in preterm labor. Her physical examination and vital signs are normal. She reports that her membranes ruptured the previous day, but labor did not start until shortly before she came to the hospital. Less than an hour after admission, a female baby weighing 2,015 g (4 lb, 7 oz), with Apgar scores of 7 at 1 minute and 9 at 5 minutes, is born. Baby Hurt's initial vital signs are

Temperature = 36.6°C (98.0°F)	Pulse = 132 beats per minute (bpm)
Respirations = 52 breaths per minute	Blood pressure = 42/36 mm Hg

You perform a Ballard examination and determine that she is 35 weeks estimated gestational age and appropriate size for gestational age. You place the baby naked in a warmed incubator and adjust the incubator temperature setting to her neutral thermal environment OR you place her on a radiant warmer bed with servocontrol set to 36.5°C skin temperature.

1. **Is the baby: ___ Well? ___ At risk? ___ Sick?**

   The baby is now 1 hour old, pink, and active. You recheck her vital signs.

2. **Indicate which value(s) is (are) abnormal.**

Normal	Abnormal	
_____	_____	**Pulse = 140 bpm**
_____	_____	**Respirations = 50 breaths per minute and unlabored**
_____	_____	**Blood pressure = 48/30 mm Hg**

   You obtain a blood glucose screening test and find that it is 45 to 90 mg%.

3. **Does this test result mean you should**

Yes	No	
___	___	**Start an intravenous line of 10% glucose?**
___	___	**Start early feedings (within 4 hours of birth)?**
___	___	**Check another screening test in an hour?**

   Next, you obtain a venous blood sample for a hematocrit. Shortly after the blood sample is sent, the laboratory technician calls and says the baby's hematocrit is 49%.

4. **Is the value: ___ Normal? ___ High? ___ Low?**

   At 2 1/2 hours of age the baby remains pink but is less active. Her vital signs now are

Temperature = 36.7° C (98.2° F)	Pulse = 140 bpm
Respirations = 68 breaths per minute, occasional grunting and nasal flaring	Blood pressure = 50/34 mm Hg
Blood glucose screening test = 45 mg%	

5. **Is the baby now: ___ Well? ___ At risk? ___ Sick?**

   The baby's lips remain pink, and the grunting and nasal flaring have not increased.

6. **What would you do for this baby now? _____**

   Shortly after the x-ray, at 3 hours of age, the baby begins retracting and has bluish lips. You give her 30% oxygen. The cyanosis does not disappear until you increase the oxygen to 45%. She becomes pink in 45% oxygen and her oxygen saturation stabilizes at approximately 90%.

   The chest x-ray shows pneumonia. The baby is now 3 hours and 15 minutes old. Her vital signs are

Temperature = 36.4° C (97.6° F)	Pulse = 150 bpm
Respirations = 70 breaths per minute with marked grunting and retracting	Blood pressure = 52/34 mm Hg
Blood glucose screening test = 25 to 45 mg%	Oxygen saturation = 88%

7. **Which of the following is now the most likely cause(s) for this baby's respiratory distress?**

_____ Respiratory distress syndrome
_____ Transient tachypnea
_____ Pneumothorax
_____ Sepsis
_____ Pneumonia

8. **What else should be done for this baby?**

Yes No

___ ___ Begin antibiotics.
___ ___ Obtain serum sodium level.
___ ___ Give sodium bicarbonate.
___ ___ Start a peripheral intravenous line.

9. **If you selected "begin antibiotics" in #8, which choice below would be appropriate?**

_____ Penicillin
_____ Gentamicin
_____ Penicillin and ampicillin
_____ Ampicillin and gentamicin
_____ None, antibiotics not indicated

By 3 1/2 hours of age, a peripheral intravenous line has been inserted with an infusion of 10% dextrose in water started and an umbilical arterial catheter inserted and connected to a heparin lock. After insertion of the umbilical arterial catheter, an x-ray is obtained to determine catheter tip location, and whether it should be repositioned.

At 4 hours of age Baby Hurt is pink in 45% oxygen. She has good muscle tone but is no longer active. Vital signs are

Temperature = 36.8°C
Respirations = 72 breaths per minute, grunting, nasal flaring, retractions
Blood glucose screening test = 45 to 90 mg%

Pulse = 145 bpm
Blood pressure = 56/36 mm Hg
Oximeter reading = 85% to 90%

The baby has received 6 mL of $D_{10}W$ and had 1.3 mL of blood removed (1.0 mL for a blood culture and 0.3 mL for an arterial blood gas). The arterial blood gas results (drawn when the baby was breathing 45% oxygen) are

PaO_2 = 42 mm Hg   pH = 7.32
$PaCO_2$ = 42 mm Hg HCO_3^- = 20 mEq/L

10. **How would you interpret the arterial blood gas results?**

PaO_2 is	_____	Low	pH is	_____	Low
	_____	Normal		_____	Normal
	_____	High		_____	High
$PaCO_2$ is	_____	Low	HCO_3^- is	_____	Low
	_____	Normal		_____	Normal
	_____	High		_____	High

11. **How would you respond to these results?** _____

Check your answers with the list near the end of the unit, immediately before the posttest.

These are the answers to the self-test questions and the sample case. Please check them with the answers you gave and review the information in the unit wherever necessary.

A1.　Well baby
　　　At-risk baby
　　　Sick baby

A2.　Normal vital signs, color, activity, feeding pattern
　　　No risk factors in the baby's prenatal and natal history
　　　Passes meconium and urinates in first 24 hours

A3.　Abnormal prenatal and/or natal history
　　　Large for gestational age or small for gestational age
　　　Preterm or post-term
　　　Previously sick baby

A4.　Any 6 of the following:
　　　• Abnormal activity (tremors, irritability, seizures, decreased tone, and/or little response to stimulation)
　　　• Abnormal heart rate (fast, slow, or irregular)
　　　• Abnormal respiratory rate (fast or slow) or pattern (episodes of apnea or difficulty breathing)
　　　• Abnormal color (cyanotic; pale, gray, or mottled; red; jaundiced)
　　　• Abnormal temperature (high, low, unstable)
　　　• Abnormal blood pressure (low blood pressure, poor capillary refill time, weak pulses)
　　　• Abnormal feeding pattern (poor feeding, abdominal distention, or recurrent vomiting)

B1.　A.　Airway: Make sure air is moving freely into the baby's lungs.
　　　B.　Breathing: Give oxygen and/or assist the baby's ventilation as necessary.
　　　C.　Circulation: Correct heart rate or blood pressure abnormalities.
　　　S.　Stabilize: Check Vital signs
　　　　　　　　　　　　　Hematocrit
　　　　　　　　　　　　　Blood glucose screening test
　　　　　– Restore them to normal or as near normal as possible.
　　　　　– Connect baby to a cardiorespiratory monitor and (usually) a pulse oximeter.
　　　　　– Decide what other problems or risk factors the baby has; evaluate and treat.

B2.　*Do not* feed a sick baby by mouth or feeding tube until the vital signs are stable.
　　　Do not bathe a sick or at-risk baby until vital signs are stable (even then a bath is unnecessary).
　　　Do not administer oxygen until you have determined a baby needs it.
　　　Do not remove a baby from oxygen, once you have determined that the baby needs oxygen.
　　　Do not perform an extensive examination until all vital signs are stable; then do a gentle gestational aging and sizing examination.
　　　Do not forget thorough hand cleansing before and after handling every baby.

B3.　Risk factors
　　　Vital signs and observations
　　　Laboratory tests

Sample Case

1.　At risk. Review her history and physical examination. You know from your assessment of the baby that she has normal vital signs, is preterm, and is appropriate size for gestational age. Therefore, this baby is not sick (vital signs normal), but she is at risk because she is preterm. The baby is also at risk because membranes were ruptured for longer than 18 hours.

2.　Her vital signs are all within normal limits (Subsection: Vital Signs and Observations).

3.　You would begin early feedings and check another blood glucose screening test in an hour (Subsection: Tests and Results).

4. Hematocrit value is normal (Subsection: Tests and Results).

5. Sick. One of the vital signs (respirations) is abnormal (tachypnea, grunting, and nasal flaring). You realize that a baby in respiratory distress cannot be fed safely by nipple, so you withhold the early feeding and plan to start an intravenous line. Remember the ABCS of Airway-Breathing-Circulation-Stabilize. Further evaluation of the baby's breathing is now important. (Airway is OK because the baby is not in acute respiratory distress, and circulation is OK as indicated by a normal pulse and blood pressure.) Possible causes for the respiratory distress include (Subsection: Vital Signs and Observatons)
    *   Respiratory distress syndrome—possible (preterm)
    *   Transient tachypnea—possible
    *   Meconium aspiration—unlikely (no meconium)
    *   Pneumonia—possible (prolonged rupture of membranes)
    *   Pneumothorax—possible
    *   Airway obstruction—unlikely given clinical course
    *   Sepsis—possible (prolonged rupture of membranes)
    *   Shock—unlikely (normal blood pressure)
    *   Hypoglycemia—unlikely (normal blood glucose)
    *   Polycythemia or anemia—unlikely (normal hematocrit)
    *   Cold baby or overheated baby—unlikely (normal temperature)
    *   Diaphragmatic hernia—unlikely but possible
    *   Tracheoesophageal fistula—unlikely but possible
    *   Congenital heart disease—unlikely but possible

    You sort through these, as shown above, and are left with 5 likely reasons for the baby's illness.
    1. Respiratory distress syndrome
    2. Transient tachypnea
    3. Pneumothorax
    4. Sepsis
    5. Pneumonia

6. Review Subsection: Vital Signs and Results
    Obtain
    *   Chest x-ray
    *   Arterial blood gas measurement
    *   White blood cell count with differential

    Attach (unless already done)
    *   Cardiorespiratory monitor
    *   Pulse oximeter

7. The chest x-ray shows pneumonia. Considering the prolonged rupture of amniotic membranes, bacterial pneumonia and sepsis are the most likely causes for the baby's respiratory distress.

8. What else should be done for this baby?

Yes	No	
x	___	Begin antibiotics (*after* obtaining a blood culture).
___	x	Obtain serum sodium level.
___	x	Give sodium bicarbonate.
x	___	Start a peripheral intravenous line

9. Antibiotics that are effective against gram-positive and gram-negative organisms should be given. The combination of ampicillin and gentamicin is an appropriate choice.

10. Review Subsection: Tests and Results

PaO_2 is low	pH is normal
$PaCO_2$ is normal	HCO_3^- is normal

11. Increase the baby's oxygen immediately, while monitoring oxygen saturation continuously. Recheck another arterial blood gas in 10 to 30 minutes.

    At 4 hours of age this baby already is quite sick. Very likely this baby will become sicker before beginning to recover, and will require several days of intensive care and several more days of convalescent care before being ready to go home.

Unit 1 Posttest

Without referring back to the information in the unit, please answer the following questions. Select the **one best** answer to each question (unless otherwise instructed). Record your answers on the answer sheet that is the last page of this book **and** on the test.

1A. An 1,800-g (4 lb), 33-week estimated gestational age baby is brought to your nursery from the delivery room. You learn an emergency cesarean section had been done because of profuse vaginal bleeding. The Apgar scores were 2 at 1 minute and 6 at 5 minutes. The baby is now 30 minutes of age and has blue lips, but is in no obvious distress. Which of the following actions should be taken within the next few minutes?

Yes   No
___   ___   Measure temperature.
___   ___   Take blood pressure.
___   ___   Measure hematocrit.
___   ___   Obtain a blood glucose screening test.
___   ___   Place the baby in oxygen.
___   ___   Connect an oximeter to the baby.

1B. By 1 hour of age the baby is in 40% oxygen, grunting and retracting slightly. His vital signs now are respirations = 60 breaths per minute, pulse = 190 beats per minute, systolic blood pressure = 26 mm Hg, temperature = 37.5°C (99.5°F) rectally. His blood glucose screening test is 40. Which of the following should have been done or should be done as soon as possible?

Yes   No
___   ___   Administer intravenous normal saline bolus, slowly.
___   ___   Give a normal saline bolus, intravenous push, quickly.
___   ___   Give an early feeding.
___   ___   Obtain an arterial blood gas sample.
___   ___   Obtain a portable chest x-ray inside the nursery.
___   ___   Attach a cardiorespiratory monitor.

1C. By 2 hours of age, the baby is still grunting and retracting in 50% oxygen in an oxyhood. A chest x-ray shows moderate respiratory distress syndrome. Laboratory results include: hematocrit = 32%, blood glucose = 20, PaO_2 = 30 mm Hg, $PaCO_2$ = 35 mm Hg, pH = 7.12, bicarbonate = 11 mEq/L. The following should have been done or would be appropriate to do now:

Yes   No
___   ___   Send blood sample for type and crossmatch.
___   ___   Give intravenous sodium bicarbonate.
___   ___   Give intravenous glucose.
___   ___   Give a bath.
___   ___   Increase baby's environmental oxygen concentration.
___   ___   Insert an umbilical arterial catheter.

1D. At 5 hours of age, the baby stops breathing for 20 seconds, turns blue, and his heart rate drops to 40 beats per minute. After stimulation, he resumes breathing and heart rate and color improve. This should be interpreted as

A. A result of his polycythemia
B. An indication the baby needs to be fed
C. Baby is getting significantly worse
D. A strong indication the baby has a congenital heart defect

2A. A baby is limp and blue at delivery with no spontaneous respirations or activity and a heart rate of 50 bpm. Her estimated weight is 1,800 g (4 lb). Within the next minute, what should be done for this baby?

Yes   No
___   ___   Begin chest compressions.
___   ___   Administer antibiotics.
___   ___   Restrict oxygen to prevent eye damage.
___   ___   Assist ventilation with anesthesia bag.

2B. By 10 minutes of age, the baby is much improved, but she still has an endotracheal tube in place, and respirations are being assisted with an anesthesia bag. Her 5-minute Apgar score was 7. She is carefully transferred to the nursery, but during the trip her endotracheal tube comes out. However, she is noted to be breathing regularly. On arrival in the nursery she is covered with vernix and dried blood and requires 50% oxygen in order to remain pink. As soon as possible, it would be important to

Yes	No	
___	___	Obtain blood pH.
___	___	Obtain a blood glucose screening test.
___	___	Bathe the baby one section at a time.
___	___	Obtain a hematocrit.
___	___	Obtain a blood pressure.
___	___	Do a detailed physical and gestational age examination.
___	___	Take the baby's temperature.

2C. At 1 hour of age, the baby is still in respiratory distress and is now requiring 70% oxygen to remain pink and maintain oximeter readings of 85% to 95%. The following information has been obtained: hematocrit 45, blood pressure 44/32, heart rate 130, respirations 60, rectal temperature 37°C (98.6°F), blood glucose screening test 45, PaO_2 65, $PaCO_2$ 65, pH 7.12, and bicarbonate 20 mEq/L. It would now be appropriate to

Yes	No	
___	___	Reintubate the baby and assist ventilation.
___	___	Give 6 mEq sodium bicarbonate (0.5 mEq/mL concentration) intravenously.
___	___	Resume chest compressions.
___	___	Obtain a portable chest x-ray inside the nursery.
___	___	Give a blood transfusion.
___	___	Give 6 mL of 10% glucose, slow intravenous push.

For each question, please make sure you have marked your answer on the test and on the answer sheet (last page in book). The test is for you; the answer sheet will need to be turned in for continuing education credit.

Unit 2   Preparation for Neonatal Transport

Objectives

In this unit you will learn

A. Which newborns may benefit from transport

B. Primary goal for preparing an infant for transport

C. How to prepare a baby for transport

D. How to support parents of transported babies

Unit 2 Pretest

Before reading the unit, please answer the following questions. Select the *one best* answer to each question (unless otherwise instructed). Record your answers on the answer sheet that is the last page in this book *and* on the test.

1A. A 1,500-g (3 lb, 5 oz) baby is born with Apgar scores of 5 at 1 minute and 9 at 5 minutes, and the decision is made to transport her to a regional perinatal center. While you are waiting for the regional center transport team to arrive, she develops severe respiratory distress with retractions and cyanosis. Which of the following should be done within the next several minutes:

Yes No
___ ___ Begin oxygen therapy.
___ ___ Transport baby to the x-ray department for a chest x-ray.
___ ___ Begin hourly tube feedings.
___ ___ Obtain an arterial blood gas.
___ ___ Check a blood sugar screening test.
___ ___ Attach a pulse oximeter.

1B. The baby continues to retract with respirations. Arterial blood gas results reveal PaO_2 = 35 mm Hg, $PaCO_2$ = 70 mm Hg, pH = 7.15, HCO_3^- = 22 mEq/L. Which of the following is most appropriate?

A. Increase inspired oxygen concentration to 100%.
B. Transport baby immediately to a regional newborn intensive care unit.
C. Intubate baby's trachea and assist ventilation with anesthesia bag and 100% oxygen.
D. Give 8 mEq sodium bicarbonate intravenously, slowly.

2. A baby is born with choanal atresia. An oral airway was immediately inserted, and the baby's vital signs are now normal and stable. Before transfer to a regional center, which of the following should be done for this baby?

Yes No
___ ___ Insert a peripheral intravenous line.
___ ___ Obtain blood culture.
___ ___ Check blood sugar screening test.
___ ___ Check blood pressure.
___ ___ Obtain electrocardiogram.

3. You suspect a baby is septic. You have obtained blood cultures and started the baby on antibiotics. Which of the following should also be done for this baby?

A. Restrict fluids
B. Electrocardiogram
C. Serum calcium level
D. Blood gas

4. A 1,200g (2 lb, 10 1/2 oz) baby is born in your delivery room. Apgar scores are 8 at 1 minute and 9 at 5 minutes, vital signs and color are normal, and there is no evidence of respiratory distress. Because of the baby's small size, plans are made to have the baby transported to a regional perinatal center. Which of these actions should be taken in your hospital by your staff before the baby is transported?

Yes No
___ ___ Administer oxygen.
___ ___ Obtain blood sugar screening test.
___ ___ Obtain chest x-ray.
___ ___ Insert umbilical arterial catheter.
___ ___ Start peripheral intravenous line.
___ ___ Feed the baby by mouth.

5. The arterial blood gas from a baby in 40% inspired oxygen shows: $PaCO_2 = 30$, $PaO_2 = 42$, pH = 7.18, $HCO_3^- = 11$. What should be done for this baby?

Yes No

___ ___ Give sodium bicarbonate.

___ ___ Provide bag-and-mask ventilation.

___ ___ Intubate and bag breathe for the baby.

___ ___ Increase the baby's oxygen.

6. A preterm baby is born after amniotic membranes have been ruptured 30 hours. The amniotic fluid is foul smelling. The baby has Apgar scores of 5 at 1 minute and 7 at 5 minutes. At 30 minutes of age the baby has a severe apneic episode that requires resuscitation. A decision is made to transport the baby to a regional perinatal center. Which of the following things should be done now, before the regional center transport team arrives?

Yes No

___ ___ Begin antibiotics, then obtain a blood culture.

___ ___ Insert an intravenous line.

___ ___ Obtain a hematocrit.

___ ___ Check a blood sugar screening test.

___ ___ Give the baby a tube feeding.

___ ___ Obtain a blood gas.

___ ___ Weigh the baby.

7. A 4,500-g (9 lb, 15 oz) baby is born to a woman with abnormal glucose tolerance. He has Apgar scores of 9 at 1 minute and 10 at 5 minutes. At 45 minutes of age, the baby has a blood sugar screening test result of 0 to 25 mg%. A peripheral intravenous infusion of 10% dextrose is started, with improvement in the baby's condition. Plans are made for neonatal transport to a regional perinatal center. Which of the following things should be done prior to transport?

Yes No

___ ___ Check blood pressure.

___ ___ Repeat blood sugar screening test.

___ ___ Give oxygen.

___ ___ Obtain a chest x-ray.

8. **True False** Babies who have experienced severe perinatal compromise require large amounts of fluid.

For each question, please make sure you have marked your answer on the test and on the answer sheet (last page in book). The test is for you; the answer sheet will need to be turned in for continuing education credit.

1. Why Are Maternal/Fetal and Neonatal Transport Important?

If maternal, fetal, or neonatal intensive care is anticipated, referral to a regional medical center may be desirable for several reasons.

- Women and/or fetuses with certain conditions may require intensive care with highly specialized monitoring and evaluation techniques for extended periods.

- Intrauterine transport is often less stressful for a baby than neonatal transport would be.

- Maternal/fetal transport allows a mother and baby to be close to each other soon after delivery.

- Maternal/fetal and neonatal transport to a regional center provide cost-effective use of highly sophisticated, expensive medical equipment and resources for patients who also require high staff-to-patient ratios.

2. What Is Neonatal Transport?

Neonatal transport occurs when an at-risk or sick newborn is transported to a regional intensive care nursery. Neonatal transport is most often accomplished by a team from a regional center that travels to the hospital of birth to transport a baby back to the regional center.

3. What Is the Goal of Preparing Any Baby for Transport?

The primary goal in preparing a baby for transport is to stabilize the infant's condition. It is more important to stabilize a baby and wait for a regional center transport team than to rush an unstable infant to a regional medical center.

 Stability of a baby's condition is far more important than speed of transport.

4. Which Babies Should Be Transported to a Regional Intensive Care Nursery?

This depends on the facilities and resources in your hospital. The medical and nursing staffs of each hospital should meet and decide which neonatal conditions can be managed locally and which need to be referred.

In general, babies with the following conditions will need care provided by a regional intensive care nursery:

- Extreme prematurity
- Malformation(s)
- Surgical conditions
- Severe, acute medical illnesses
- Complex, long-term medical needs

5. What Is the Minimum Preparation for *Every* Baby for Transport?

A. Check Vital Signs
- Temperature
- Respiratory rate
- Heart rate
- Blood pressure

B. Perform Laboratory Tests
- *Blood sugar screening test*: important for nearly all babies
- *Hematocrit*: important for most babies
- *Blood gases*: important for babies requiring supplemental oxygen, or requiring respiratory support, even if supplemental oxygen is not being used
- *Other tests*: according to the baby's condition and the reason transport is needed

C. Establish a Fluid Line

This may be a peripheral intravenous (IV) line, umbilical venous catheter, and/or umbilical arterial catheter, depending on the baby's condition. A fluid line is important for 2 reasons.
- Infusion of fluids during transport
- Emergency medications may be needed

D. Call the Regional Center and Discuss the Baby's Condition
- *History*: pregnancy complications, risk factors, Apgar scores, baby's approximate weight and gestational age, early neonatal course, etc
- *Present status*: physical examination, including a description of any malformations, vital signs, oxygen and ventilation requirements, etc
- *Laboratory values*: blood sugar screening test, hematocrit, blood gases, and/or chest x-ray, etc
- *Need for further special treatment*

There will be some babies you recognize immediately as requiring transport. It is reasonable to call the regional center to activate the transport process before all information is available. When additional information becomes available, a follow-up telephone call is usually helpful for a detailed discussion of the infant's condition.

E. Discuss the Baby's Condition With the Parents; Document This and Obtain a Signed Permit for Transport and Complete Forms Required to Be Compliant With HIPAA (Health Insurance Portability and Accountability Act)

F. Obtain Complete Copies of the Charts
- Mother's chart
- Baby's chart

G. Obtain Blood Samples
- 10 mL mother's blood, if possible (purple-top tube, containing anticoagulant, is preferable, but a clot tube is acceptable)
- 10 mL cord blood, if available

H. Obtain Copies of Any X-rays of the Baby

I. Continue Optimum Supportive Care

Once a transport has been arranged, it is essential that optimum care be delivered while waiting for the transport team to arrive. It is your responsibility to ensure that the baby maintains adequate oxygenation, temperature, blood pressure, and stable metabolic status during this time.

To provide optimum supportive care means that you should check the baby's vital signs and certain laboratory tests repeatedly, perhaps as often as every 30 minutes. Chest x-rays and/or other tests may also need to be repeated, depending on the baby's condition.

 Care given during the first few hours after birth is every bit as important to a baby's outcome as care given during days or weeks at a regional intensive care nursery.

Some sick babies may need additional tests and procedures to be stabilized and prepared for transport. These have been discussed in the previous units. Material in this book will also help you to decide which specific tests and procedures each individual baby requires.

Self-Test

Now answer these questions to test yourself on the information in the last section.

A1. What is the minimum preparation needed for every baby who will be transported?

_____

_____

_____

_____

_____

_____

_____

_____

_____

A2. What is the primary goal in preparing a baby for transport?

_____

A3. Least at least 3 groups of babies that are likely to need care at a regional intensive care nursery.

_____

_____

_____

Check your answers with the list near the end of the unit, immediately before the posttest. Correct any incorrect answers and review the appropriate section in the unit.

6. How Should You Prepare Babies With Special Problems for Transport?

Some information given below is *only* in this section. It is found nowhere else in the Perinatal Continuing Education Program books.

Respiratory Distress

Obtain These Tests or Procedures	Look Particularly for These	Do This Before Transport
Chest x-ray	• Pneumothorax	• Perform needle aspiration and/or insert chest tube if baby is in significant respiratory distress and/or blood gases or oxygen saturation are abnormal.
Arterial blood gases	• Low PaO_2	• Increase oxygen. • Consider baby may have a pneumothorax.
	• High $PaCO_2$	• Consider bag-and-mask ventilation or endotracheal intubation and assisted ventilation. • Consider baby may have a pneumothorax.
	• Low pH	• If $PaCO_2$ is high, consider assisted ventilation. • If $PaCO_2$ and bicarbonate are low, determine and treat the cause of the acidosis and consider giving sodium bicarbonate.
Blood cultures	• Any baby with respiratory distress may be infected, with the infection being a cause of the respiratory distress.	• Consider obtaining blood cultures and beginning antibiotics.
Consider giving surfactant	• RDS by x-ray and baby has endotracheal tube in place.	• Whether to give surfactant before transport depends on many factors. Lung compliance changes rapidly after surfactant administration, thus requiring close attention to ventilator management. Discuss with regional center staff.

Severe Perinatal Compromise

Obtain These Tests or Procedures	Look Particularly for These	Do This Before Transport
Arterial blood gases	• Low PaO_2	• Increase inspired oxygen concentration.
	• Low pH	• If $PaCO_2$ and bicarbonate are low, consider giving sodium bicarbonate.
Note:	Kidneys and heart of a baby who experienced an episode of hypoxia and/or acidosis may not be able to handle a large amount of fluid.	• Restrict IV fluids, but beware of the possible development of hypoglycemia. • Consider you may need to increase glucose concentration in the IV fluid.

Shock

Obtain These Tests or Procedures	Look Particularly for These	Do This Before Transport
Blood pressure	• Low blood pressure	• Look for the cause of shock and treat appropriately. • If no cause is apparent, or if you suspect blood loss, give blood volume expander (10 mL/kg, slowly).
Blood gases	• Low pH	• Venous blood gas may be used to check pH. • If there is any evidence of respiratory distress, however, obtain an arterial blood gas.

Suspected Sepsis

Obtain These Tests or Procedures	Look Particularly for These	Do This Before Transport
Blood cultures		• Start antibiotics immediately after obtaining cultures. *Do not wait for culture results.* • Use antibiotics that combat gram-positive and gram-negative organisms.
Blood gases	• Low pH	• Venous blood gas may be used to check pH. • If there is any evidence of respiratory distress, however, obtain an arterial blood gas.
Consider CBC	• Low WBC count: ratio of immature to total polymorphs of >0.2	• Obtain cultures and start antibiotics, if not done earlier.

Seizures

Obtain These Tests or Procedures	Look Particularly for These	Do This Before Transport
Determine blood glucose	• Low	• Give glucose.
Determine blood calcium	• Low	• Give calcium.
Lumbar puncture	• High WBC count	• Culture spinal fluid and treat baby with antibiotics. • If infection with gram-negative organism is suspected, consider giving cephalosporin or other antibiotic that crosses into the cerebrospinal fluid. • Use "meningitic" doses of ampicillin. • Give anticonvulsant immediately.*
	• Bloody	• Suspect birth trauma.
Birth asphyxia or cause unknown		• Give anticonvulsant immediately.*

*Give phenobarbital 20 mg/kg, intravenously. The dose may be repeated to achieve suppression of seizures, but be prepared to ventilate the baby if respiratory depression occurs.

40

Suspected Congenital Heart Disease (CHD)

Obtain These Tests or Procedures	Look Particularly for These	Do This Before Transport
Blood pressure (check measurements in all 4 extremities)	• Hypotension	Babies with congenital heart disease (CHD) may have hypotension or hypertension, depending on the type and severity of the defect. *Hypotension* may be present due to poor cardiac output.
	• Hypertension	*Hypertension* may be present from obstructed blood flow that can occur with certain defects (eg, coarctation of the aorta).
	• Differences among extremities	Blood pressure may vary in different extremities. If blood pressure measurements from all 4 extremities vary significantly, that information may be helpful in making a diagnosis and determining therapy.
Arterial blood gas (ABG)	• Acidosis	*Metabolic acidosis* may be present because of poor cardiac output, in which case treatment with dopamine and/or sodium bicarbonate may be indicated. *Respiratory acidosis* may be present due to hypoventilation, in which case intubation and assisted ventilation may be indicated.
	• Hypoxemia	Certain cardiac abnormalities cause *cyanotic* CHD. Other defects cause *acyanotic* (no cyanosis due to the defect itself) heart disease. With cyanotic heart disease, a baby's PaO_2 will rarely be >50–60 mm Hg, even if the baby is breathing 100% oxygen. For these babies an intravenous infusion of prostaglandin E_1 (PGE_1) may be recommended. There are very few situations where PGE_1 therapy will make a baby's CHD symptoms worse for the few hours that may be required to make a definitive diagnosis. For some unstable babies, PGE_1 therapy may dramatically improve their condition by dilating the ductus arteriosus and thereby permitting blood to flow to the lungs or the systemic circulation (depending on the nature of the cardiac lesion). ***Consult with regional center experts when CHD is suspected.*** If PGE_1 therapy is recommended, follow these guidelines. *Route*: Give by continuous IV infusion. Use a large central vein. Infuse into the umbilical vein, with the catheter tip located above the diaphragm. If that is not available, infusion through a peripheral vein is acceptable, but may cause cutaneous flushing around the infusion site. *Dose and rate*: Give 0.05–1.0 mcg/kg/minute. Usually 0.05 mcg/kg/minute is adequate and is associated with fewer side effects. *Preparation*: This drug is supplied in 500 mcg/mL vials. Dilute 1 vial with either D_5W or normal saline (NS), according to this chart.

D_5W or NS	Infusion Rate to Give 0.05 mcg/kg/minute	
	mL/kg/minute	mL/kg/hour
100 mL	0.01	0.6
200 mL	0.02	1.2

Side effects: Fever and apnea are commonly seen soon after initiation of PGE_1 therapy. **Be prepared, BEFORE infusion of PGE_1 is started, to assist the baby's ventilation.**

Congenital Malformations

Condition	Do This Before Transport
All conditions listed below, follow 1 and 2 at right.	**1. Do not feed the baby.** **2. Maintain hydration with IV fluids.**
Choanal atresia	• Place oral airway. Intubate baby if respiratory distress does not resolve with airway placement.
Diaphragmatic hernia	• Insert nasogastric tube ($\geq$8F) and suction intermittently OR if a Replogle tube is available, use it and suction continuously. • Keep baby positioned at 45° angle (head up). • If baby requires assisted ventilation, intubate. Do *not* use bag-and-mask ventilation.
Intestinal obstruction	• Insert nasogastric tube ($\geq$8F) and apply intermittent suction OR if a Replogle tube is available, use it and apply continuous suction.
Meningomyelocele	• Place the baby on his/her abdomen. • If the sac is ruptured, keep it covered with warm sterile saline dressings. Use smooth, non-adhering dressing material; do *not* use gauze. • Avoid using latex products because they may cause sensitization.
Pierre Robin anomaly (small mandible with respiratory distress)	• Insert a 10F or 12F catheter through the nose and into the posterior pharynx. This will break the suction that pulls the tongue into the airway, causing respiratory distress. • Place the baby on his/her abdomen.
Ruptured omphalocele or gastroschisis	• Give IV fluids (1/2 NS) at a rate of 8–10 mL/kg/hour. • Place the baby's lower body (*below* defect) in a bowel bag (used to contain intestines during adult abdominal surgery) to keep urine and meconium away from the defect; place the baby and first bowel bag into another sterile bowel bag, to enclose the defect and baby up to the axilla. This will minimize heat loss and trauma to the exposed organs, and allow visualization of the defect. A small quantity (about 5–10 mL) of normal saline may be put in the second bowel bag to keep the intestines moist. • Do *not* wrap intestines with gauze. Gauze, even if it seems soft, can damage the delicate surface of the organs. It may also act as a wick to draw away fluid and protein that may weep from the exposed surface of the organs. • Insert nasogastric tube ($\geq$8F) and suction intermittently OR if a Replogle tube is available, use it and suction continuously. • Position baby on his/her side.
Tracheoesophageal fistula	• Suction pouch with size $\geq$8F feeding tube. • Keep baby positioned at 45° angle (head up).

Sample Case 1

Use the material in the unit, *and in the previous unit,* to help you answer these sample cases.

Baby Johns is born at 32 weeks by maternal dates, weighing 1,360 g (3 lb), and begins grunting and retracting almost from the moment of birth. The baby has a 1-minute Apgar score of 9 but by 5 minutes requires oxygen by mask held to his face to stay pink. The baby is transferred in a warm incubator to the nursery while receiving 60% inspired oxygen concentration. Nothing else is known about the baby's history.

1. **How would you classify this baby?**

    ___ Well?   ___ At risk?   ___ Sick?

2. **What would you do immediately for this baby?**

    _____

    _____

    You find that the blood sugar screening test is 45 to 90 mg%, blood pressure is 22/18 mm Hg, hematocrit is 31%, and oxygen saturation is 92%.

3. **What should be done now for this baby?**

    _____

    _____

4. **What 2 things would you do next?**

    _____

    The blood pressure is now 36/28 mm Hg, and the blood glucose screening test is now 90 mg%. The chest x-ray is consistent with respiratory distress syndrome. The arterial blood gas result in 60% inspired oxygen is

    $$PaO_2 = 62 \text{ mm Hg} \qquad pH = 7.27$$
    $$PaCO_2 = 45 \text{ mm Hg} \qquad HCO_3^- = 20 \text{ mEq/L}$$

5. **What would you do now for Baby Johns?**

Yes	No	
___	___	**Increase the baby's inspired oxygen.**
___	___	**Decrease the baby's inspired oxygen.**
___	___	**Give normal saline.**
___	___	**Give 25% glucose intravenous push.**

    At 40 minutes of age, the baby's vital signs are

    > Temperature = 37.0°C (98.6°F) (radiant warmer servocontrol)
    > Pulse = 152 beats/minute
    > Respirations = 72 breaths/minute
    > Blood pressure = 38/30 mm Hg

    It has been decided that Baby Johns needs to be transferred to the regional intensive care nursery.

6. **What else should be done to prepare this baby for transport?**

    _____

    _____

    You continue this optimal supportive care (frequent blood glucose screening tests, temperature control, frequent blood pressure measurements, arterial blood gases, and assist baby's ventilation, as necessary) and consultation with regional center staff until the transport team arrives.

Check your answers with the list near the end of the unit, immediately before the posttest.

Sample Case 2

Full-term, appropriate size for gestational age Baby George, born after an uncomplicated pregnancy, is pink, active, and irritable at 18 hours of age. His vital signs have been stable. The baby has nursed well at the breast and has urinated, but has not passed meconium since birth. His abdomen has become distended and slightly tense. He vomited the last feeding.

1. **How would you classify this baby?**

   ___ Well?   ___ At risk?   ___ Sick?

2. **What would you think of as possible causes for the abdominal distension?**

   _____

   _____

3. **Of these things, which one is the most likely cause?**

   _____

4. **What should be done to evaluate this baby?**

   _____

   _____

The baby's vital signs are

    Temperature = 37.0°C (98.7°F)   Blood pressure = 66/38 mm Hg
    Pulse = 156 beats/minute   Blood glucose screening test = 90 mg%
    Respirations = 48 breaths/minute, unlabored

5. **How should this baby be fed?**

   _____

The laboratory calls and says that Baby George's hematocrit is 52%.

6. **How should this be treated?**

   _____

20 mL of gastric fluid have been suctioned through the nasogastric tube.

7. **What should be done with this?**

   _____

The baby remains pink and active. The abdomen remains distended but is less tense. The mother and father come into the nursery and rock their baby. The vital signs are now

    Temperature = 37.0°C (98.7°F)   Blood pressure = 71/40 mm Hg
    Pulse = 148 beats/minute   Blood glucose screening test = 90 mg%
    Respirations = 48 breaths/minute

The abdominal x-ray shows dilated loops of bowel consistent with an intestinal obstruction.

The decision is made to transfer this baby to the regional intensive care nursery. The regional center staff is contacted to arrange to transport Baby George.

8. **What else should be done to prepare this baby for transport?**

   _____

   _____

Check your answers with the list near the end of the unit, immediately before the posttest.

Subsection: Caring for Parents of Transported Babies
Objectives

In this section you will learn

A. Why it is important for parents to be involved in the care of their sick or at-risk baby

B. Some ways to encourage emotional attachment of parents to their sick or at-risk baby

C. Special considerations when providing information to parents about their baby's condition

D. Special considerations for the hospitalized mother following transport of her baby

Involvement of the parents* is an extremely important aspect of the care of a sick or at-risk baby. Early, frequent, and close parent contact with a sick newborn is essential to develop a strong, healthy bond between parents and their baby. There are several things you can do for the family of every transported baby that will aid this attachment process.

1. How Do You Encourage Emotional Attachment With the Baby?

Allow and encourage parents to enter the nursery to visit their baby before the transport team arrives. This can be done without any interruption in the care being given to the baby. In fact, it is important not to change a baby's care (unless the baby's condition changes) during parental visits.

There are a few simple techniques that can be used to help foster the development of emotional ties between parent and child prior to transport.

- *Seeing and touching the baby.* All of the equipment should be explained, but lengthy details are rarely needed at this time. Most parents focus immediately on their infant; some parents need more help. Have them stroke the baby's palm. Even the smallest and sickest babies can usually grasp a parent's finger.

- *Quick-developing or digital color snapshot of the baby.* Discuss this and obtain permission from the parents before taking a photograph. All equipment should remain attached to the infant when the picture is taken. Most parents see past the apparatus and focus on their baby.

- *Hand and/or foot print(s) of the baby for the parents to keep.*

Whether a baby is a perfectly formed but tiny preterm infant or a full-term baby with a malformation, he or she is not the "ideal" healthy baby every parent imagines and hopes for. Parents need to establish strong bonds of affection and commitment to their child during the stressful, rocky period of illness.

Parents of a baby with a malformation should be encouraged to see and touch their infant. What a parent imagines is almost always far worse than the baby's real condition. Parents need an honest and accurate understanding of their baby's condition so that they can begin to deal with the real problems that confront their baby and themselves. Efforts to protect the parents by heavy sedation of the mother or by restricting contact with the baby are not helpful.

The attitude of "don't get involved because the baby will probably die" is also not realistic or helpful. Most sick babies do not die. Most preterm infants, given proper care, live and have no residual problems. Most term sick babies also live and do well. Even if a baby dies, grieving is more easily accomplished and resolved when parents have close and caring ties

---

*"Parents" indicates mother and father or, in the case of an absent father, a second person of the mother's choosing.

with their baby than when they feel distant, isolated, or unimportant to their baby.

Regardless of the medical condition, parents need help as they begin the process of getting to know the unique characteristics, needs, and personality of their baby. Even parents who have long planned and waited for the birth of this baby are often fearful to undertake the process of emotional attachment when confronted with a sick baby. Your understanding and assistance can be of tremendous value to the parents at this time.

In addition, many fears and misunderstandings typically accompany the birth of a sick baby. Family members and parents may be inappropriately judgmental about whose "fault" it is that the baby is sick. It is the responsibility of the medical and nursing staff to explore with the parents their feelings, correct misunderstandings, and facilitate the process of parents becoming acquainted with their newborn.

2. What Should You Tell the Family About the Baby's Condition?

Parents should have a clear understanding of their baby's condition. Frequently, repeated discussions and explanations are necessary for parents to gain this understanding.

Serious conditions should be presented honestly and realistically. It is not necessary, however, to discuss all of the *possible* complications. Many of these problems will not develop, but once the possibility has been raised, it is difficult to erase it from a parent's mind. Doubts may linger long after the danger has passed. For example, once a parent has been told that a preterm infant may be "brain damaged" or "retarded" without any real evidence of this, it is not uncommon for parents years later to treat their normal child as abnormal, or to watch anxiously for any sign that the child is mentally handicapped. This may be because parents of even mildly ill babies often feel their baby will die. In other words, parents often expect the worst and may need repeated reassurance about their baby's actual condition.

When a baby is being transported, it is helpful for the referring hospital staff to accompany regional center transport team members when they discuss the baby's condition with the parents. The referring hospital staff can then reinforce what the transport team has said and correct any misunderstanding that may develop after the team has left.

3. How Do You Provide for Parents' Special Needs?

If possible, it may be helpful for the mother to have a private room so she is not confronted by roommates feeding and cuddling healthy newborns.

Visiting hours should be relaxed so that parents can spend as much time together as they wish. Between employment, family responsibilities, and visiting the regional center to see their sick baby, it is often impractical if not impossible for fathers to comply with visiting regulations. Close communication between parents is important for their relationship during this stressful time; it is also important for the father to relay accurate information about the baby to the mother. Often fathers will want to "protect" mothers from hearing about worsening illness or complications that have occurred. While this protective feeling is understandable, the mother should be fully informed.

After babies have been transferred to a regional center, mothers often need reassurance about their baby's condition at unpredictable times, such as when seeing a baby product advertisement on television or having a sleepless night. Talking with someone or calling the regional center intensive care nursery may be helpful at these times.

Summary

- Encourage parents to see and touch their baby. If needed, help them to make this contact.
- Provide picture and/or footprints of their baby, according to parents' wishes and available resources.
- Provide repeated, realistic explanations of the baby's condition.
- Give "bad news" only if, and when, complications develop.
- Know what information the transport team has given the parents.
- Consider providing the mother with a private room.
- Relax visiting policies.
- Provide emotional support to both parents and to other family members.

How Do You Arrange for a Baby to Be Transported?

A. Call the Regional Center

In the space below, write the hospital name, telephone number, and any special instructions you would use to make a neonatal referral and arrange for transport of a newborn.

B. Discuss the Baby's History and Condition With the Regional Center Staff

C. Prepare the Baby (section 5A–I for all babies and section 6A–G for babies with special problems)

D. Continue Optimum Supportive Care

These are the answers to the self-test questions and the sample case. Please check them with the answers you gave and review the information in the unit wherever necessary.

A1. Minimal preparation for every baby includes
- Check vital signs.
- Obtain blood glucose screening test, hematocrit, blood gases, and/or other tests, as indicated by baby's condition.
- Establish a fluid line.
- Call the regional center and discuss the baby's condition.
- Obtain a sample of mother's blood and cord blood (if available).
- Obtain complete copies of the mother's chart and the baby's chart.
- Obtain copies of any x-rays of the baby.
- Talk with the parents, document the discussion, and have a transport permit and other necessary forms signed.
- Continue optimum supportive care.

A2. Stabilize the baby's condition and vital signs.

A3. Babies with any of the following conditions:
- Extreme prematurity
- Malformation(s)
- Surgical conditions
- Severe, acute medical illnesses
- Complex, long-term medical needs

Note: Referral is often indicated for other babies too.

Answers to Sample Case 1

1. Baby Johns has abnormal respirations and is, therefore, sick.

2. Check vital signs, blood glucose screening test, hematocrit, arterial blood gas. Attach a pulse oximeter.

3. Unit 1, Subsection: Vital Signs and Observations and Unit 2, section 6
- Insert an umbilical venous catheter.
- Give 15 mL (10 mL/kg) of normal saline, slowly, no faster than 1 to 2 mL/minute.
- Send a blood sample for type and crossmatch.

4. Recheck the blood pressure. Obtain a chest x-ray.

5. Yes No
Yes	No	
____	x	Increase the baby's inspired oxygen (Unit 1, Subsection: Tests and Results).
____	x	Decrease the baby's inspired oxygen.
____	x	Give normal saline (Unit 1, Subsection: Vital Signs and Observations).
____	x	Give 25% glucose intravenous push (Unit 1, Subsection: Tests and Results).

6. Unit 2, section 5, each of the following:
- Obtain 10 mL of the mother's blood.
- Obtain 10 mL of cord blood, if available.
- Obtain complete copies of both the mother's chart and the baby's chart.
- Obtain copies of the baby's x-rays.
- Discuss the baby's condition with the parents, document this discussion, and have a permit for transport and any other necessary forms signed. Answer any questions the parents have, and encourage them to see and touch their baby.

You should continue to monitor vital signs, blood glucose screening tests, arterial blood gases, and oximeter readings, and provide supportive care and respond to any changes in the baby's condition while you await the arrival of the transport team.

Answers to Sample Case 2

1. The baby has abnormal feeding pattern and therefore is sick.

2. Unit 1, Subsection: Vital Signs and Observations
   - Sepsis
   - Gastrointestinal obstruction
   - Necrotizing enterocolitis

3. Gastrointestinal obstruction: The baby is pink, is active, has normal vital signs, has nursed well, and has no risk factors for sepsis. Sepsis is a possibility, but is less likely than gastrointestinal obstruction in this baby. Necrotizing enterocolitis occurs most often in sick, preterm infants. This baby is term and was not previously sick, making gastrointestinal obstruction a more likely cause.

4. Continue to look in Unit 1, Subsection: Vital Signs and Observations
   - Check the baby's vital signs.
   - Check blood glucose screening test and hematocrit.
   - Check arterial or venous blood gas measurement (done to look for a low pH due to metabolic acidosis).
   - Consider obtaining cultures and beginning antibiotics.
   - Pass a size 8F or larger nasogastric tube and connect to low, constant suction, or leave the tube open to air and, at frequent intervals, use a syringe to aspirate stomach contents.
   - Obtain chest and abdominal x-ray.

5. This baby should not be fed by mouth or tube, but should have a peripheral intravenous line started.

6. Unit 1, Subsection: Tests and Results. The hematocrit is normal and, therefore, requires no treatment.

7. The gastric fluid may be discarded, but the volume should be recorded. Electrolytes are contained within the gastric juices. If significant volumes continue to be aspirated, the baby's serum electrolytes will need to be checked and perhaps sodium chloride may need to be added to the intravenous fluids to keep the serum electrolytes within the normal ranges.

8. Unit 2, section 5
   - Obtain 10 mL of the mother's blood.
   - Obtain 10 mL of cord blood, if available.
   - Obtain complete copies of both the mother's chart and the baby's chart.
   - Obtain copies of the baby's x-rays.
   - Discuss the baby's condition with the parents, document this discussion, and have a permit for transport and any other necessary forms signed. Answer any questions the parents have, and encourage them to see and touch their baby.

You have already made the specific preparations necessary for the transport of a baby with an intestinal obstruction (Unit 2, section 6G). Be sure to continue to suction intermittently from the gastric tube. You should continue to monitor vital signs, provide supportive care, and respond to any changes in the baby's condition while you await the arrival of the transport team.

Unit 2 Posttest

Without referring back to the information in the unit, please answer the following questions. Select the **one best** answer to each question (unless otherwise instructed). Record your answers on the answer sheet that is the last page in this book *and* on the test.

1. The arterial blood gas from a baby with respiratory distress shows a normal PaO_2 value, a high $PaCO_2$ value, and low pH value. What would you do for this baby?

   A. Increase the baby's inspired oxygen concentration.
   B. Give sodium bicarbonate.
   C. Assist ventilation.
   D. Decrease the baby's inspired oxygen concentration.

2. **True   False**   A blood gas measurement is important for a baby suspected of being septic.

3. Which of the following tests is (are) particularly important for a baby who has had a seizure, but otherwise appears well?

   Yes   No
   ___   ___   Determine blood glucose.
   ___   ___   Determine blood calcium.
   ___   ___   Do a lumbar puncture.

4. A baby was born in shock due to blood loss and had a mean blood pressure of 22 mm Hg. This was treated with normal saline. The mean blood pressure is now 40 mm Hg. What would you do now for this baby?

   Yes   No
   ___   ___   Crossmatch the baby's blood.
   ___   ___   Check serum calcium.
   ___   ___   Give phenobarbital.
   ___   ___   Check hematocrit.

5. A 3,500-g (7 lb, 11 1/2 oz) baby is born meconium-stained, with Apgar scores of 0 at 1 minute and 1 at 5 minutes. He required intubation and full resuscitation. At 25 minutes of age, he is breathing well on his own and has normal vital signs, but requires 40% oxygen to remain pink. Because of possible post-resuscitation complications, the decision was made to have the baby transported to a regional perinatal center. What should be done prior to transport?

   Yes   No
   ___   ___   Start an intravenous infusion.
   ___   ___   Give IV fluid bolus.
   ___   ___   Obtain a blood gas.
   ___   ___   Obtain a chest x-ray.
   ___   ___   Check a blood sugar screening test.
   ___   ___   Perform a lumbar puncture.

6. A 1,000-g (2 lb, 3 oz) baby is born and has Apgar scores of 5 at 1 minute and 8 at 5 minutes. When in the nursery, the baby is pink and vital signs are as follows: respirations = 40 breaths/minute and unlabored, heart rate = 130 beats/minute, blood pressure = 40/18 mm Hg, and temperature = 35°C (95.0°F). Because of the baby's small size, neonatal transport to a regional perinatal center has been arranged. Which of the following should be done prior to transport?

   Yes   No
   ___   ___   Give volume expander.
   ___   ___   Give oxygen.
   ___   ___   Warm the baby.
   ___   ___   Obtain hematocrit.
   ___   ___   Obtain chest x-ray.
   ___   ___   Begin intravenous line.
   ___   ___   Feed the baby by mouth.
   ___   ___   Bathe the baby.

7. An 1,800-g (4 lb) baby is born with Apgar scores of 6 at 1 minute and 7 at 5 minutes. In the delivery room, the baby is noted to grunt and retract. The baby is placed in 60% oxygen and taken to the nursery. Plans are made to have the baby transported to a regional perinatal center. While an intravenous line is being started, the baby suddenly turns blue and respiratory distress increases. What should be done for this baby?

Yes   No

___   ___   Obtain a skull x-ray.

___   ___   Obtain a blood gas.

___   ___   Increase the environmental oxygen.

___   ___   Give blood volume expander.

___   ___   Listen for breath sounds.

___   ___   Obtain a chest x-ray.

8A. A 1,500-g (3 lb, 5 oz) baby is born with Apgar scores of 5 at 1 minute and 9 at 5 minutes. She develops severe respiratory distress at 2 hours after birth and the decision is made to transport her to the regional perinatal center. The baby continues to retract severely and color becomes blue. Which of the following should be done within the next several minutes:

Yes   No

___   ___   Begin oxygen therapy.

___   ___   Transport baby to the x-ray department for chest x-ray.

___   ___   Begin hourly tube feedings.

___   ___   Obtain arterial blood gas.

___   ___   Check a blood glucose screening test.

8B. The baby continues to retract and remains cyanotic. Arterial blood gas results reveal

$$PaO_2 = 35 \text{ mm Hg}$$
$$PaCO_2 = 70 \text{ mm Hg}$$
$$pH = 7.18$$
$$HCO_3^- = 25 \text{ mEq/L}$$

Which of the following is most appropriate?

A. Increase inspired oxygen concentration to 100%.

B. Place baby in transport incubator and transport immediately to a regional perinatal center.

C. Insert a chest tube.

D. Intubate baby's trachea and assist ventilation with anesthesia bag and 100% oxygen.

For each question, please make sure you have marked your answer on the test and on the answer sheet (last page in book). The test is for you; the answer sheet will need to be turned in for continuing education credit.

Unit 3

Direct Blood Pressure Measurement

Objectives

In this unit you will learn the

A. Difference between direct and indirect blood pressure monitoring

B. Reasons for direct blood pressure monitoring

C. Equipment needed for direct blood pressure monitoring

D. Interpretation of blood pressure waveforms

Unit 3 Pretest

Before reading the unit, please answer the following questions. Select the *one best* answer to each question (unless otherwise instructed). Record your answers on the answer sheet that is the last page in this book *and* on the test.

1. A damped pressure tracing may be caused by each of the following *except*

    A. Air bubbles in the tubing
    B. Hypotension
    C. Severe anemia
    D. A clot at the tip of the umbilical catheter

2. **True   False**   Special intravenous tubing is needed for direct blood pressure monitoring.

3. **True   False**   A narrowed pulse pressure may indicate certain congenital heart defects.

4. **True   False**   The normal range of direct blood pressure measurements is different than the normal range for indirect blood pressure measurements.

5. **True   False**   When a direct blood pressure monitoring waveform shows slow decrease in pressure during diastole, it may be an indication of increased systemic vascular resistance.

6. The transducer for direct blood pressure measurement should be level with the

    A. Baby's heart
    B. Electronic monitor
    C. Umbilical catheter
    D. Intravenous infusion pump

7. Direct blood pressure measurement is used for each of the following reasons *except*

    A. Continuous blood pressure monitoring
    B. Increased accuracy of the measurements
    C. Obtaining information about a baby's cardiac status
    D. Measurement of acid-base balance

For each question, please make sure you have marked your answer on the test and on the answer sheet (last page in book). The test is for you; the answer sheet will need to be turned in for continuing education credit.

1. What Are the 2 General Types of Blood Pressure Monitoring?

A. Indirect Blood Pressure Measurement

Indirect measurement is the typical way in which blood pressure is measured. An inflatable cuff is wrapped around an extremity. The cuff is then inflated to a pressure somewhat higher than the anticipated blood pressure. Manual palpation or a mechanical device is used to detect changes in arterial flow as the cuff is deflated (Book II: Neonatal Care, Blood Pressure).

B. Direct Blood Pressure Measurement

Direct blood pressure measurement occurs when the measuring device is connected to a catheter inserted directly into an artery. An umbilical artery or a peripheral artery may be used as the monitoring site.

2. How Are Direct Blood Pressure Measurements Made?

An arterial catheter is connected to special tubing that resists changes in pressure. This non-distensible tubing is used to transmit the arterial pressure at the catheter tip to a transducer. The transducer converts the mechanical pressure of blood in an artery into an electrical signal. The electrical signal is displayed on a cardiac monitor oscilloscope. The resulting pattern is the blood pressure waveform.

3. Why Is Direct Blood Pressure Measurement Used?

Direct monitoring is used in sick babies who have an arterial catheter in place. It is especially important for unstable babies. The 3 primary advantages of direct monitoring are

*   It allows continuous blood pressure monitoring.

*   It gives the most accurate form of blood pressure measurement.

*   Waveform shape may suggest certain clinical conditions.

4. What Equipment Is Needed for Direct Blood Pressure Monitoring?

General points regarding direct blood pressure monitoring are presented here; details of the technique are covered in the skill unit. The following equipment is needed for direct blood pressure monitoring:

A. Arterial Catheter

In babies, an umbilical arterial catheter is most commonly used. Occasionally a small catheter is placed in one of the peripheral arteries, usually a radial artery, and then connected to the appropriate monitoring equipment.

B. Electronic Monitor With Oscilloscope

This monitor has one channel that allows continuous cardiac (electrocardiogram [ECG]) monitoring and another channel for blood pressure monitoring. It has a calibrated screen where the blood pressure waveform, as well as a digital readout of the systolic, diastolic, and mean blood pressures, are displayed.

C. Non-distensible Tubing

This connects the arterial catheter and the transducer. It is made of stiff plastic and is sometimes called high-pressure tubing.

D. Transducer

Several brands of disposable transducers are available.

E. Transducer Cable

This connects the transducer with the electronic monitor. Sometimes the transducer and cable are a single unit.

F. Intravenous (IV) Pump

This pump should be able to deliver a low volume of fluid (<1 mL/hour). It should also be able to deliver fluid continuously, rather than in pulses. Usually this is a syringe pump.

G. Intravenous Solution

To obtain continuous blood pressure readings, the system must remain open between the catheter and the transducer. This significantly increases the risk of clot formation within the catheter, unless a continuous infusion of IV fluid is maintained.

Normal saline will cause less sludging of blood in a catheter than will a glucose solution; however, small babies may receive excessive sodium and insufficient glucose if normal saline is used to help keep the catheter patent. Calculate the requirements of your patient (Book II: Neonatal Care, Hypoglycemia and IV Therapy).

Whichever IV solution is selected, heparinizing it with 0.5 to 1.0 units of heparin per milliliter of IV solution and infusing it at a rate of at least 0.5 mL/hour is generally recommended for arterial lines.

H. Mechanism to Hold Transducer at the Level of the Baby's Heart

Sometimes the transducer is mounted on an IV pole with a holder that may be raised or lowered as the baby's position is changed. Most commonly, however, transducers are designed to rest on the bed alongside the baby.

Self-Test

Now answer these questions to test yourself on the information in the last section.

A1. Indirect blood pressure measurement uses an _____ _____ wrapped around the baby's arm or leg, while direct blood pressure measurement uses a _____ inserted into an _____.

A2. What are the 3 primary reasons for using direct blood pressure monitoring?

_____

_____

_____

A3. **True** **False** A continuous infusion should be given through an umbilical arterial catheter when it is being used for continuous blood pressure monitoring.

A4. **True** **False** Non-distensible tubing is an optional piece of equipment for continuous direct blood pressure monitoring.

A5. **True** **False** An intravenous pump that delivers fluid in regular, tiny pulses is the preferred type of pump to use with a direct blood pressure monitoring arterial catheter.

Check your answers with the list near the end of the unit. Correct any incorrect answers and review the appropriate section in the unit.

5. What Are Normal Neonatal Blood Pressure Ranges?

Figures 3.1, 3.2, and 3.3 show the normal and abnormal ranges of blood pressure for babies of different birth weights and at different gestational and postmenstrual ages. These are the same graphs that were first presented in Book II: Neonatal Care, Blood Pressure.

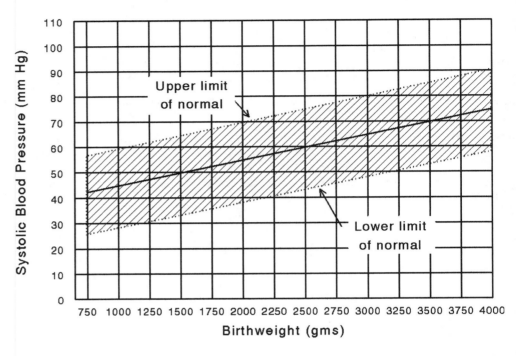

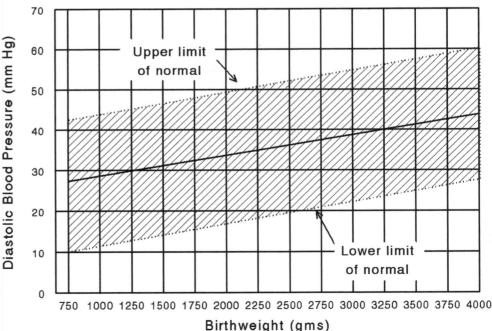

Figure 3.1. Blood Pressure During First Day After Birth

The blood pressure graphs on these 2 pages were created from data published in Zubrow AB, Hulman S, Kushner H, Falkner B. Determinants of blood pressure in infants admitted to neonatal intensive care units: a prospective multicenter study. *J Perinatol*. 1995;15:470.

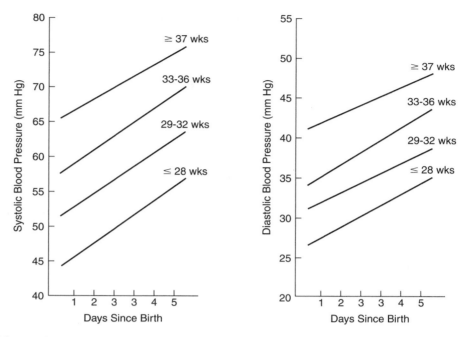

Figure 3.2. Blood Pressure for Babies of Different Gestational Ages During First 5 Days After Birth

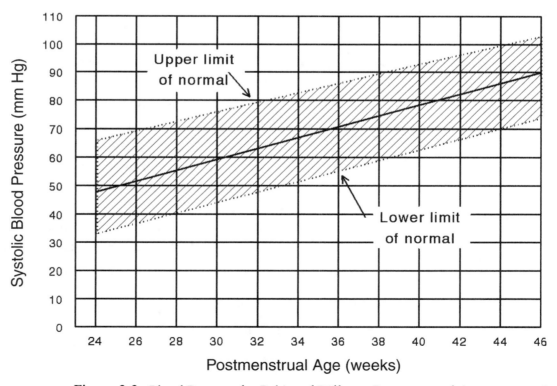

Figure 3.3. Blood Pressure for Babies of Different Postmenstrual Ages

6. How Do You Interpret Blood Pressure Waveforms?

A. Blood Pressure Waveform: Normal Configuration

Figure 3.4 shows a normal newborn blood pressure waveform, as it appears in relation to a cardiac monitor (ECG) tracing.

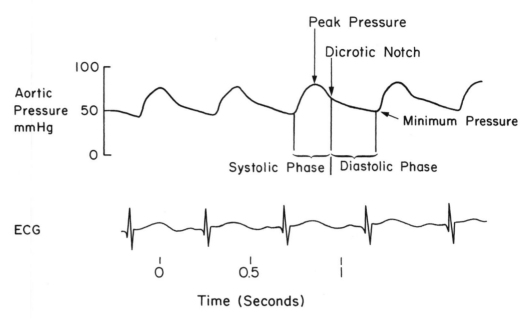

Figure 3.4. Arterial Waveform

The shape of the pattern corresponds with events happening within the heart. These are described as follows:

- *Systolic phase:* time during which the heart is ejecting blood
- *Peak pressure:* the highest point during systole (systolic pressure)
- *Dicrotic notch:* point of closure of the aortic valve
- *Diastolic phase:* time during which the heart is filling with blood
- *Minimum pressure:* the lowest point during diastole (diastolic pressure)
- *Pulse pressure:* the difference between peak and minimum pressures
- *Mean pressure:* the average pressure of the complete cardiac cycle

The key segments to recognize are the sharp rise during systole, the dicrotic notch, and the slower fall in pressure during diastole.

In addition to displaying the blood pressure waveform, nearly all monitors have digital displays of continuous readings of systolic, diastolic, and/or mean arterial pressure.

B. Abnormal Configuration

1. Damped waveform

The most common cause of an abnormal pressure waveform is a damped tracing in which the waveform "flattens out." Usually the systolic pressure will seem to be decreased and the diastolic pressure will seem to be increased, causing little change in the mean arterial pressure. These changes may be subtle or they may be more dramatic, leading to an almost flat line for a pressure tracing. A damped waveform with subtle changes can be recognized by the disappearance of the dicrotic notch.

A damped tracing may be caused by

a. *Air bubbles within the tubing or at the transducer:* These air bubbles may be very tiny. Careful inspection of the full length of the tubing and all connections is required. If air bubbles are found they should be flushed from the system while taking care not to infuse any into the baby. Flush the tubing and transducer by

   - Turning the stopcock off to the baby
   - Opening the transducer to air
   - Flushing the IV fluid through the transducer and out the port open to air

b. *Kink in the tubing:* This is a rare occurrence but should be considered whenever a waveform is damped.

c. *Hypotension:* A baby in shock may also seem to have a damped waveform. Always be sure to check the blood pressure values by indirect means and assess the baby's clinical condition.

d. *Clot at the tip or within the lumen of the catheter:* This is the most common reason for a damped tracing. If this is the suspected cause of a damped waveform, aspirate blood from the catheter. Then slowly flush the catheter with 0.5 to 1.0 mL of flush solution. Reopen the system between the catheter and the transducer. If the waveform remains damped, and no other cause for a damped tracing can be found, the catheter needs to be removed.

 If a waveform is damped due to a suspected clot at the tip or within the lumen, the catheter needs to be removed and replaced with a new one.

2. Abnormally shaped waveform

   Waveforms of particular shape, or changes in a baby's waveform, may suggest abnormal cardiac status. These findings are usually subtle and should be considered only *suggestive* of the corresponding problem.

Finding	Possible Cause
• Slow pressure increase during early systole	• Poor left ventricular contractility • Aortic stenosis
• Slow pressure decrease during diastole	• Increased systemic vascular resistance
• Rapid pressure decrease during diastole	• Left-to-right shunting, such as from a patent ductus arteriosus

C. Abnormally Wide or Narrow Pulse Pressure

Pulse pressure is the difference between peak systolic and minimum diastolic pressures. Wide or narrow pulse pressure may *suggest* certain cardiac abnormalities. A change in pulse pressure may *suggest* the development of certain problems, such as a pneumothorax or pneumopericardium, which may affect cardiac function.

Reliable normal values of pulse pressure in newborns have not been defined. A pulse pressure less than 10 mm Hg, however, is generally considered too narrow.

A pulse pressure significantly greater than the value of the diastolic pressure is generally considered too wide. For example, a systolic pressure of 60 mm Hg and a diastolic pressure of 20 mm Hg gives a pulse pressure of 40 mm Hg, which is significantly greater than the diastolic pressure.

Pulse Pressure	Possible Cause
• Narrowed	• Coarctation of the aorta
	• Pneumothorax
	• Pneumopericardium or hemopericardium
	• Aortic stenosis
	• Hypoplastic left heart
	• Shock (cardiogenic, septic, or hemorrhagic)
	• Heart failure
• Widened	• Patent ductus arteriosus
	• Aortopulmonary window
	• Arterial-venous fistula
	• Truncus arteriosus
	• Hyperthyroidism
	• Aortic regurgitation

These waveform findings are only suggestive of the abnormalities listed and must be considered together with other clinical and diagnostic findings. Consult your regional center if you have any questions about a baby's cardiac status.

Self-Test

Now answer these questions to test yourself on the information in the last section.

B1. A damped waveform may be caused by

Yes	No	
___	___	Hypotension
___	___	Air bubbles in the tubing
___	___	Patent ductus arteriosus
___	___	Clot at the catheter tip

B2. **True** **False** The pulse pressure is the same as the mean pressure.

B3. **True** **False** The lowest point of the waveform indicates the diastolic pressure.

B4. List 2 possible causes of a *narrowed* pulse pressure.

_____

_____

B5. List 2 possible causes of a *widened* pulse pressure.

_____

_____

Check your answers with the list near the end of the unit. Correct any incorrect answers and review the appropriate section in the unit.

These are the answers to the self-test questions. Please check them with the answers you gave and review the information in the unit wherever necessary.

A1.   Indirect blood pressure measurement uses an *inflatable cuff* wrapped around the baby's arm or leg, while direct blood pressure measurement uses a *catheter* inserted into an *artery*.

A2.   The 3 primary advantages of direct blood pressure monitoring are
   • Provides most accurate form of blood pressure measurement
   • Allows continuous measurement of blood pressure
   • Waveform shape may aid in the diagnosis of certain clinical conditions

A3   True

A4.   False   Only non-distensible tubing allows accurate transmission of pressure between the catheter and the transducer without being "lost" in the elasticity of regular intravenous tubing.

A5.   False   An intravenous pump that delivers a low volume of fluid continuously, rather than in pulses, is the preferred type of pump for direct blood pressure monitoring.

B1.   Yes   No
   _x_   ___   Hypotension
   _x_   ___   Air bubbles in the tubing
   ___   _x_   Patent ductus arteriosus
   _x_   ___   Clot at the catheter tip

B2.   False   The pulse pressure is the difference between peak (systolic pressure) and minimum (diastolic pressure) pressures. Mean blood pressure is the average pressure of the complete cardiac cycle.

B3.   True

B4.   Any 2 of the following are possible causes of a *narrowed* pulse pressure:
   • Coarctation of the aorta
   • Pneumothorax
   • Pneumopericardium or hemopericardium
   • Aortic stenosis
   • Hypoplastic left heart
   • Shock (cardiogenic, septic, or hemorrhagic)
   • Heart failure

B5.   Any 2 of the following are possible causes of a *widened* pulse pressure:
   • Patent ductus arteriosus
   • Aortopulmonary window
   • Arterial-venous fistula
   • Truncus arteriosus
   • Hyperthyroidism
   • Aortic regurgitation

Unit 3 Posttest

Without referring back to the information in the unit, please answer the following questions. Select the *one best* answer to each question (unless otherwise instructed). Record your answers on the answer sheet that is the last page in this book *and* on the test.

1. A damped pressure tracing may be caused by each of the following *except*
   A. A kink in the tubing
   B. Air bubbles in the tubing
   C. Hypertension
   D. Hypotension

2. The dicrotic notch represents the
   A. End of diastole
   B. Closure of the aortic valve
   C. Beginning of systole
   D. Presence of a patent foramen ovale

3. **True   False**   When continuous direct blood pressure monitoring is used, an intravenous solution should be infused continuously through the catheter.

4. **True   False**   A slow decrease in pressure during diastole may indicate a patent ductus arteriosus with left-to-right shunting.

5 **True   False**   In babies, only umbilical arterial catheters can be used for direct blood pressure measurement.

6. Pulse pressure is the
   A. Highest pressure during systole
   B. Difference between the systolic and diastolic pressures
   C. Lowest pressure necessary to generate a pulse
   D. An artificial calculation derived from the systolic blood pressure and heart rate

7. All of the following are used for direct blood pressure measurement, *except*
   A. Electronic monitor
   B. Umbilical arterial catheter
   C. Transducer
   D. Blood pressure cuff

For each question, please make sure you have marked your answer on the test and on the answer sheet (last page in book). The test is for you; the answer sheet will need to be turned in for continuing education credit.

Skill Unit

Transducer Blood Pressure Monitoring

This skill unit will teach you the principles of continuous electronic blood pressure monitoring.

Study this skill unit, then attend a skill practice and demonstration session. You will learn how to apply the principles learned in this unit to the specific equipment used in your hospital.

To master the skill, you will need to demonstrate correctly each of the following steps, using the specific equipment available in your hospital:

1. Assemble equipment.
2. Set up continuous infusion.
3. Flush tubing and transducer with infusion fluid.
4. Connect tubing to "baby's" (manikin's) arterial catheter.
5. Level transducer with "baby's" heart.
6. Zero monitor.
7. Set alarms.
8. Measure "baby's" blood pressure.

Perinatal Performance Guide
Using Transducer Blood Pressure Monitors

Actions	**Remarks**

Preparing the Equipment

1. Collect the equipment.
   - Electronic monitor
   - Non-distensible (high-pressure) tubing
   - Transducer
   - Transducer cable
   - Infusion pump that can deliver less than 1 mL/hour in continuous flow (not pulses)
   - Heparinized intravenous (IV) solution
   - 3-way stopcock
   - Adjustable-height clamp to hold transducer at the level of the baby's heart (optional)

   The baby should have an arterial catheter already in place. A 3-way stopcock should already be attached to the end of the catheter.

   In general, syringe pumps are used.

   This is usually pharmacy prepared.

   Many transducers are designed to rest on the baby's bed, next to the baby. Know the requirements of the transducer you are using.

2. Assemble the equipment.

   Most transducer kits come preassembled with tubing for the IV infusion → transducer → stopcock → non-distensible tubing already connected in the proper sequence. If yours do not, connect the pieces in that sequence.

3. Set up the continuous infusion.

   Any appropriate IV solution heparinized with 0.5 to 1.0 units/mL may be used. See section 4G in the unit.

4. Flush the heparinized IV solution through the IV tubing, transducer, stopcock, and non-distensible tubing.

   As an additional safeguard, non-distensible tubing that has an air-bubble filter incorporated into it is available. Know the features of the tubing used in your hospital.

   Be sure to clear the tubing of ALL air bubbles, including very tiny bubbles.

   If the tubing is flushed slowly, air bubbles are generally less of a problem. Also, hold the transducer so the exit to the non-distensible tubing is upright. This will help ensure that the transducer fills completely and no air bubbles are trapped in a corner of it.

5. Connect the non-distensible tubing to the stopcock that is at the end of the baby's arterial catheter.

6. Use a syringe on the third port of the stopcock (the stopcock that is connected to the arterial catheter) to draw blood into the catheter to be sure there is a brisk blood return before beginning to infuse fluid through the catheter.

   There is no need to pull blood into the syringe or even to fill the catheter with blood. You just need to see a flash of blood in the catheter and observe that the catheter can be aspirated easily.

Actions	Remarks

Preparing the Equipment (continued)

7. Turn the stopcocks so they are open between the baby's arterial catheter and the IV fluid, as shown in the figure below.

   Double-check to be sure there are no air bubbles in the tubing.

8. Begin infusion of the heparinized IV fluid. Infusion at a rate of at least 0.5 mL/hour is generally recommended.

   Neither this infusion rate nor the IV fluid used is designed to fulfill a baby's fluid requirements, but to keep the catheter patent. Keep track of the volume infused because even this low infusion rate can provide a significant volume for small babies.

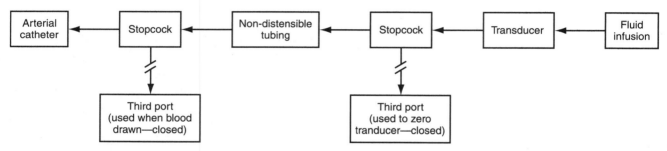

Configuration During Infusion: System Open Between IV Fluid and Arterial Catheter

Calibrating the Blood Pressure Monitor

9. With the baby supine, level the transducer with the baby's heart. Use the baby's midaxillary point to approximate the level of the heart. In most cases this may be accomplished by simply putting the transducer flat on the bed next to the baby.

   In some cases, it may be useful to tape the transducer to a disposable diaper and place that next to the baby. This will keep the transducer flat and raise it *slightly* off the bed, to the midaxillary level of the baby's chest.

   Sometimes transducers are clamped to a pole beside the bed and, if so, should be clamped at a point level with the baby's midaxillary area.

   However the transducer is positioned, it is important that the position relative to the baby remain constant. Changing the transducer level compared to the baby can result in false readings.

Actions   **Remarks**

Calibrating the Blood Pressure Monitor (continued)

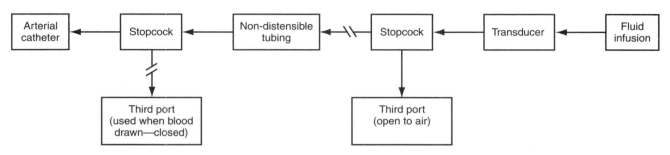

Configuration During Calibration: System Closed to Arterial Catheter (Baby), Open Between Transducer and Air

10. Zero the monitor.

    - Open the transducer to atmospheric pressure. This is done by turning the system off to the baby and open between the transducer head and air, as shown in the figure above.

    - Adjust the oscilloscope so that the blood pressure reads zero.   In most cases, this is accomplished simply by pressing a "zero" button on the monitor screen.

    Note: Some monitors need to be calibrated to both zero and a higher number, usually 100 mm Hg.   Be sure you know the requirements of the specific equipment used in your hospital.

11. Begin to monitor the baby.
    - Close the system to atmospheric pressure and reopen it between the IV infusion and the baby's arterial catheter.   The system should again be configured the same as shown in the figure on page 74.

    - Cap the port that was open to atmospheric pressure with a syringe or sterile cap.

    - Check again to be sure no air bubbles have entered the tubing.   Sometimes air enters the stopcock, and then into the tubing, when the stopcock is opened to air during calibration.

    - Check to be sure the monitor is set for a scale appropriate to neonatal blood pressure values.   Most monitors have 2 or 3 pressure scales that may be used. Generally, the 0 to 100 mm Hg scale is used for babies. If a different scale is used, the waveform may sometimes, depending on a baby's blood pressure, appear to be off the screen.

Actions	**Remarks**

Measuring the Baby's Blood Pressure

Actions	**Remarks**
12. Set the alarm limits appropriate to the baby's blood pressure. If the baby is hypotensive initially, readjust the alarm limits as the blood pressure is corrected.	Determine if the alarm limits on your monitor can be set for systolic/diastolic and/or mean blood pressure. Then set the alarm limits 5 to 10 mm Hg higher and 5 to 10 mm Hg lower than the baby's blood pressure reading.
13. Observe the character of the pressure waveform. Determine if the waveform is a damped or an undamped tracing.	If the waveform is damped, investigate the cause. Review section 6B(1) in the unit.
14. Read and record the baby's blood pressure. This may be read from the screen or the digital readout.	Usually the baby's systolic, diastolic, and mean arterial pressures are recorded (eg, 65/45 MAP 53). If a digital readout is not available, only the systolic and diastolic pressures can be read from the waveform tracing on a calibrated monitor screen.
15. Make regular, routine examinations of the tubing to be sure no air bubbles have entered the system.	If an air bubble(s) is found, remove it from the system.
16. Check the baby's blood pressure periodically by indirect measurement with an inflatable cuff.	Direct and indirect blood pressure readings should correlate very closely.
17. Periodically repeat steps 9 through 11 to calibrate the monitor.	The transducer setup is commonly calibrated 2 to 3 times a day, whenever the disposable transducer and tubing are changed, and whenever there is a question about waveform quality.

Unit 4   Exchange, Reduction, and Direct Transfusions

Objectives

In this unit you will learn

A. Why exchange, reduction, and direct transfusions are performed

B. What type of donor blood is used

C. The effects of anticoagulants on donor blood

D. How to prepare donor blood

E. How exchange, reduction, and direct transfusions are performed

F. How to monitor the baby for potential complications

Unit 4 Pretest

Before reading the unit, please answer the following questions. Select the *one best* answer to each question (unless otherwise instructed). Record your answers on the answer sheet that is the last page in this book *and* on the test.

1. **True**   **False**   Blood glucose screening test should be checked immediately after any exchange transfusion.

2. **True**   **False**   When an umbilical arterial catheter is used in an exchange transfusion, it is used only to withdraw blood from the baby.

3. **True**   **False**   No baby should have more than one exchange transfusion.

4. **True**   **False**   Packed red blood cells (hematocrit >70%) of appropriate group and type should be used for an exchange transfusion.

5. A reduction exchange transfusion is different from an exchange transfusion for hyperbilirubinemia because
   A. A larger volume of blood is exchanged.
   B. Infectious complications are more likely to occur.
   C. Blood is not given.
   D. Rebound hypoglycemia is more likely to occur.

6. The tip of a venous catheter used to perform an exchange transfusion should be in the
   A. Left atrium of the heart
   B. Femoral vein
   C. Abdominal aorta
   D. Inferior vena cava

7. What is the preferred age of donor blood used for an exchange transfusion?
   A. 1 to 10 days old
   B. 10 to 15 days old
   C. 15 to 20 days old
   D. Age of the blood is not an issue

8. **True**   **False**   A term 3,000-g (6 lb, 6 oz) baby with tachypnea, a blood glucose screening test of 25 mg/100 mL, and a venous hematocrit of 68% should receive a reduction exchange transfusion.

9. **True**   **False**   Phototherapy lights should be used after every exchange transfusion for hyperbilirubinemia.

10. **True**   **False**   All preterm infants should be transfused with packed red blood cells if their hematocrits are less than or equal to 25%.

11. **True**   **False**   Capillary blood from a heel stick sample is the preferred way to test a baby's hematocrit.

12. Which of the following is a possible sign of anemia in a stable, growing preterm baby?
   A. Rapid weight gain
   B. Hypoglycemia
   C. Hyperbilirubinemia
   D. Tachypnea

13. Which of the following babies is at *lowest* risk for polycythemia?
   A. 30-week baby appropriate for gestational age
   B. 40-week baby small for gestational age
   C. 43-week baby appropriate for gestational age
   D. 38-week baby of a diabetic mother

14. An 1,800-g (4 lb) preterm baby is severely anemic and requires a transfusion of packed red blood cells. How much blood would you give?

    A. 10 mL

    B.   18 mL

    C.   36 mL

    D. 162 mL

For each question, please make sure you have marked your answer on the test and on the answer sheet (last page in book). The test is for you; the answer sheet will need to be turned in for continuing education credit.

Exchange Transfusions in the Management of Hyperbilirubinemia

Note: This section will discuss exchange transfusions for hyperbilirubinemia only. Exchange transfusions for other purposes (eg, sepsis, disseminated intravascular coagulation, or metabolic disorders) require other techniques and types of donor blood.

1. What Is an Exchange Transfusion?

An exchange transfusion entails withdrawing a small amount of blood from a baby and replacing it with an equal amount of donor blood, then repeating this process many times until most of the baby's blood has been removed and replaced with donor blood.

Routes of exchange include

- An umbilical venous catheter (UVC) alone may be used to perform an exchange transfusion.

- Umbilical venous and arterial catheters may be used simultaneously, with blood withdrawn through the arterial catheter and infused though the venous catheter.

- Blood may also be withdrawn through an umbilical arterial catheter (UAC), peripheral arterial catheter (PAC), or UVC and infused through a peripheral intravenous (PIV) line.

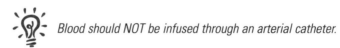 *Blood should NOT be infused through an arterial catheter.*

2. Why Is an Exchange Transfusion Done?

There are 3 purposes for an exchange transfusion in the treatment of severe hyperbilirubinemia.

- Remove bilirubin.

- Remove sensitized red blood cells and replace them with non-sensitized red blood cells (for hyperbilirubinemia due to blood group incompatibility).

- Remove circulating antibodies (for hyperbilirubinemia due to blood group incompatibility).

Note: Refer to Book II: Neonatal Care, Hyperbilirubinemia to determine *when* exchange transfusion(s) should be used to treat hyperbilirubinemia.

3. What Type of Donor Blood Is Used?

A. Hyperbilirubinemia Due to Rh Incompatibility
- Rh-negative red blood cells of the baby's blood group (A, B, AB, or O) resuspended in plasma of the same ABO group as the infant

- Type O, Rh-negative red blood cells resuspended in type AB plasma

B. Hyperbilirubinemia Due to ABO Incompatibility

- Group O, Rh-compatible red blood cells resuspended in plasma of the same ABO group as the infant, or in group AB plasma

4. How Should the Blood Be Preserved?

The freshest available and most suitable blood should be used. It is important to know the anticoagulant used and how that substance may affect the baby. Citrate phosphate dextrose adenine (CPDA-1) is the anticoagulant most often used and can cause any of the following problems:

- *Hypocalcemia:* Citrate binds the electrolyte calcium, therefore, calcium replacement may be necessary during and/or shortly after an exchange transfusion. Calcium replacement should be given if the baby shows signs of hypocalcemia. Signs of hypocalcemia include jitteriness, seizures, or apnea.

  If the baby is symptomatic, 1 to 2 mL of calcium gluconate in 10% (100 mg/mL) concentration is *given very slowly* through a UVC, with the tip located in the inferior vena cava. Calcium gluconate in 10% concentration may be diluted with sterile water for injection to 5% and 2 to 4 mL given, as described.

  The baby's heart rate must be electronically monitored continuously. The calcium infusion is *stopped immediately* if the baby's heart rate begins to slow. (See the skill unit for the details of calcium administration.)

- *Hypoglycemia:* Babies with Rh isoimmune disease often have hyperactive insulin-secreting cells. In addition, any baby may develop "rebound hypoglycemia" once the exchange transfusion has been completed, due to the high concentration of dextrose in CPDA-1–preserved blood. Any baby receiving an exchange transfusion should have blood glucose screening tests checked immediately after the exchange and hourly for several more hours.

- *Acidosis or alkalosis:* CPDA-1–preserved blood has a pH range of 7.5 to 7.6 at the beginning of storage but may fall to 7.0 or lower as storage time lengthens. Most infants can metabolize the preservative without difficulty. With citrate-preserved blood, alkalosis may develop as citrate is metabolized in the liver to form bicarbonate. Bicarbonate, of course, is a buffer used to counteract acidosis. The resulting metabolic alkalosis may persist for several days.

- *Hyperkalemia:* For an exchange transfusion in babies, use of CPDA-1–preserved donor blood that is 10 or fewer days old is recommended. Blood stored for more than 10 days may develop potassium levels that are dangerously high for babies.

5. How Much Blood Is Used for an Exchange Transfusion?

Generally, 180 mL of donor blood for every kilogram (1,000 g) of the baby's weight is used for an exchange transfusion. When 180 mL/kg is used, it is called a 2-volume exchange because a baby's average blood volume is 90 mL/kg. A 2-volume exchange transfusion will remove and replace 85% to 90% of an infant's original blood.

Immediately after a 2-volume exchange, the baby's bilirubin level can be expected to be one third to one half the pre-exchange bilirubin level.

6. What Else Is Done to Prepare Blood for an Exchange Transfusion?

A. Determine the Hematocrit

The hematocrit of adult blood used for an exchange transfusion may be too low for a baby because

- Newborn hematocrits are generally higher than adult hematocrits.
- The anticoagulant added to the adult blood dilutes it and further lowers the hematocrit.
- Babies with Rh or ABO incompatibility may be anemic due to the rapid breakdown of their red blood cells.

Donor blood with a hematocrit value of 45% to 55% should be used for neonatal exchange transfusions. Most blood banks can prepare blood with appropriate hematocrit by mixing packed cells and plasma in the necessary ratio.

B. Warm the Blood

The blood should be warmed using a commercially available blood warmer with

- Constant temperature readout
- Adjustable thermostat
- Alarm system to prevent overheating the blood

Note: Radiant warming devices or older immersion warmers without the characteristics listed above are dangerous and should *not* be used.

Summary of Preparation Steps

The following 5 steps should be taken to prepare donor blood for an exchange transfusion:

1. Select the appropriate blood group and Rh type.

2. Know the anticoagulant used and the age of the blood.

3. Calculate the volume of blood to be exchanged.

4. Know the hematocrit of the blood prepared by the blood bank.

5. Warm the blood with a commercial device that has the necessary safety features.

Self-Test

Now answer these questions to test yourself on the information in the last section.

A1. What are 4 possible problems with the use of citrate phospate dextrose adenine–preserved blood?

_____

_____

_____

_____

A2. The hematocrit of donor blood used in an exchange transfusion should be _____.

A3. **True   False**   Blood is best warmed under a radiant warmer.

A4. Immediately after a 2-volume exchange transfusion, the baby's bilirubin will be _____ to _____ the level it was before the exchange.

A5. Identify whether each of the following may be used to withdraw and/or infuse blood.

	Withdraw		Infuse	
	Yes	No	Yes	No
Umbilical arterial catheter	___	___	___	___
Peripheral arterial catheter	___	___	___	___
Umbilical venous catheter	___	___	___	___
Peripheral intravenous line	___	___	___	___

Check your answers with the list near the end of the unit, immediately before the posttest. Correct any incorrect answers and review the appropriate section in the unit.

7. How Is an Exchange Transfusion Performed?

Although the precise details of the techniques for exchange transfusion are given in the skill unit, several points are especially important and will be mentioned here. These are

A. Methods of Exchange

1. <u>Pull-Push Method</u>: The pull-push method, in which a small volume of the baby's blood is withdrawn (pulled) through a UVC, followed by an equal volume of donor blood infused (pushed) through the UVC to the baby. This pull-push cycle is repeated until the exchange transfusion is completed.

2. <u>Continuous Method</u>: With the continuous method the baby's blood is withdrawn through one line and, simultaneously, an equal amount of donor blood is infused through a second line.

   Blood may be withdrawn from a UVC or arterial catheter, or from a PAC, and given, in equal volume, through a PIV line. The baby's blood may also be withdrawn through an arterial catheter and donor blood infused simultaneously through a UVC, if the UVC is above the liver with the tip in the inferior vena cava.

   Although the continuous method has the advantage that it can be performed more quickly, it has the disadvantage that catheters and syringes are more likely to become clotted with blood. If clots develop, the UVC, PIV line, and/or syringe(s) need to be replaced.

Regardless of the exchange method, blood should *not* be infused through an artery. The risk of tissue damage from the accidental infusion of emboli due to air bubbles or tiny blood clots is much greater when blood is infused through an artery than when it is infused through a vein.

For either exchange method, withdrawal and infusion should be done slowly and steadily to avoid sudden shifts in the baby's blood pressure. Sudden shifts in blood pressure have been associated with intraventricular bleeding in newborns, particularly in preterm infants. Withdrawal rate and infusion rate no faster than 2 to 3 mL/kg/minute are recommended.

Summary of Exchange Routes

Pull-Push Method: Blood is alternately withdrawn and infused in small increments through a UVC.

Continuous Method: Blood is withdrawn through one line and simultaneously infused through another. Appropriate withdrawal and infusion routes are

Withdrawal Route	Infusion Route
UAC $\longrightarrow$	UVC or PIV
PAC $\longrightarrow$	UVC or PIV
UVC $\longrightarrow$	PIV

B. Catheter Position

Ideally, the tip of a UVC should be in the inferior vena cava, as confirmed by x-ray.

If this position cannot be achieved and bilirubin levels are considered to be dangerously high, an exchange transfusion can be performed through a UVC when the catheter tip is still in the umbilical vein and has not yet entered the vena cava, but there is a somewhat greater risk of liver damage. In this case, the catheter should be inserted only 1 to 2 cm and, preferably, used only to withdraw blood. Sclerosing drugs such as calcium probably should not be infused through a catheter in this position.

 Regardless of UVC location, blood flow should be obtained easily from the catheter before starting any exchange transfusion.

If a UAC is used to withdraw blood, it should be inserted and positioned as outlined in Book II: Neonatal Care, Umbilical Catheters. A peripheral IV in any location may be used to infuse blood.

C. Keep Blood Mixed

The actual process of exchanging the baby's blood for donor blood takes approximately 1 to 2 hours to complete, depending on the volume of blood and exchange method used. During this time, it is important to mix the donor blood several times to prevent further separation of the red blood cells from the plasma. Mixing the blood is done by gently agitating the donor blood bag by hand every 10 to 15 minutes.

If the blood is allowed to settle during the procedure, the baby will receive mostly plasma at the end of the exchange transfusion. This may cause the baby to have a low post-exchange hematocrit.

D. Record Keeping

- *A minimum of 2 people is required for a pull-push exchange transfusion.* After the UVC is inserted, the second person is required to keep precise records of the blood exchanged and medications, if any, given to the baby.

- *Three people are generally required for a continuous exchange:* one to withdraw the baby's blood, one to infuse the donor blood, and one to keep records.

With either method, each small increment of blood withdrawn and given is recorded, as well as a "running total" of all blood removed from and given to the baby.

Precise, detailed records are extremely important to avoid accidentally overloading the baby with fluid, or leaving the baby in a hypovolemic state at the end of the exchange.

8. Will a Baby Ever Need More Than One Transfusion?

Most babies with hyperbilirubinemia do *not* require an exchange transfusion. Refer to Book II: Neonatal Care, Hyperbilirubinemia to determine *if and when* a particular baby needs an exchange transfusion.

For a baby with hyperbilirubinemia severe enough to require one exchange transfusion, it is possible for the baby to require more than one exchange. An exchange transfusion will not remove all of the baby's circulating bilirubin.

Rebound hyperbilirubinemia may occur after an exchange is completed. The baby's bilirubin level should be checked every 4 to 6 hours after an exchange.

 Phototherapy lights should always be used after every exchange transfusion for hyperbilirubinemia.

9. What Are the Potential Complications of an Exchange Transfusion?

An exchange transfusion is an important, but invasive, therapeutic measure for a baby with severe hyperbilirubinemia. With careful preparation and careful monitoring of the baby's cardiac and metabolic status, the complications listed below can be minimized or avoided.

Potential Complications of Exchange Transfusions

Possible Complications	Means to Monitor/Prevent Complications
Vascular	
• Formation of air or blood emboli	• Use careful technique when infusing through a UVC. • Do *not* infuse through a UAC or PAC.
• Thrombosis	• Be sure there is adequate blood return from the catheter and do not leave the catheter in place longer than necessary.
• IV infiltration	• If a PIV line is used to infuse donor blood, observe the site carefully throughout the infusion.
Cardiac	
• Arrhythmias	• Monitor continuously with electronic heart rate monitor. • Check electrolytes if heart rate pattern changes.
• Volume overload, volume depletion	• Keep precise records of blood given to and taken from the baby. • Obtain blood pressure measurements at least every 15 minutes during the exchange.
• Cardiorespiratory arrest	• Continuously monitor baby with electronic heart rate monitor. • Keep resuscitation equipment at bedside.
Clotting	
• Catheter clotted	• Be aware that this is more likely to happen when an arterial catheter is used to withdraw blood during a continuous exchange. Periodically flush the UAC or PAC with a small volume of heparinized saline.

Potential Complications of Exchange Transfusions (continued)

Possible Complications	Means to Monitor/Prevent Complications
Metabolic • Hypocalcemia (low blood calcium level) • Hypoglycemia (low blood glucose level) • Hyperkalemia (high blood potassium level) • Hypernatremia (high blood sodium level) • Rebound hyperbilirubinemia	• Obtain blood studies for glucose, calcium, potassium, sodium, and bilirubin after the exchange transfusion and as indicated by the baby's condition.
Infectious • Sepsis • Serum hepatitis • Cytomegalovirus (CMV) • Human immunodeficiency virus (HIV)	• Maintain sterile technique throughout the exchange transfusion. • Blood bank screens blood donors carefully, tests blood. • Blood bank screens blood donors carefully, tests blood. • Blood bank screens blood donors carefully, tests blood.
Miscellaneous • Mechanical injury to donor cells • Perforation of the inferior vena cava • Hypothermia • Tanning (injury from over-heating) of the red blood cells • Anemia • Thrombocytopenia	• Use only a commercial blood warmer that has passed quality inspection for temperature control and alarm system. • This is rare, but if resistance is met when a UVC is inserted, it should not be forced further. • Warm the blood to 37°C (98.6°F). • Maintain temperature control of the baby during the procedure. • Do *not* warm the blood under a radiant warmer. Be sure the temperature of a commercial blood warmer does not go above 38.0°C (100.4°F). • Be sure the blood bank measures the hematocrit of the donor blood. • Mix the blood frequently during the procedure. • Check a post-exchange platelet count. Neither red blood cell components nor plasma contain viable platelets.

Self-Test

Now answer these questions to test yourself on the information in the last section.

B1. **True** **False** If an umbilical venous catheter is used to withdraw a baby's blood for an exchange transfusion, the donor blood should be infused through an umbilical arterial catheter.

B2. List at least 2 possible *cardiac* complications of an exchange transfusion.

_____

_____

B3. Following an exchange transfusion for hyperbilirubinemia, a baby's bilirubin level should be checked every _____ to _____ hours.

B4. List at least 3 possible *metabolic* complications of an exchange transfusion.

_____

_____

_____

Check your answers with the list near the end of the unit, immediately before the posttest. Correct any incorrect answers and review the appropriate section in the unit.

Reduction Exchange Transfusions in the Management of Polycythemia

1. What Is a Reduction Exchange Transfusion?

A reduction exchange transfusion, also called a partial exchange transfusion, is the process of withdrawing a calculated amount of the baby's blood and replacing it with an equal amount of normal saline.

2. Why Is a Reduction Exchange Transfusion Done?

Reduction exchange transfusions are performed to reduce the number of red blood cells in babies with polycythemia.

A. What Is Polycythemia?

Polycythemia is a condition in which a baby has more red blood cells than normal, with a resulting increase in hematocrit. When the hematocrit is higher than approximately 65%, blood flow may become sluggish.

Sluggish blood flow may, in turn, cause poor tissue perfusion. The organs most affected by sluggish flow may vary from baby to baby, leading to a wide range of possible problems.

Some babies with hematocrits between 65% to 70% will not have any of the signs listed below, but almost all babies with hematocrits 70% or above will show one or more of the following:

- Plethora (ruddy appearance)
- Cyanosis
- Lethargy
- Poor feeding
- Respiratory distress
- Congestive heart failure
- Tremors
- Seizures
- Hypoglycemia
- Hyperbilirubinemia

B. How Is Polycythemia Diagnosed?

Blood drawn from a vein or artery should be used to measure a baby's hematocrit. Capillary blood, or blood obtained when a heel stick is done, should *not* be used. While capillary blood, from a fingerstick, will provide accurate results in adults, this is *not* true for newborns.

Blood obtained from heel sticks in newborns can give falsely high hematocrit values due to venous stasis. Alternatively, if the heel is squeezed excessively to collect the blood sample, interstitial fluid may dilute the sample and give falsely low hematocrit values.

Polycythemia should not be diagnosed from a newborn capillary (heel stick) blood sample. Only blood drawn from a vein or artery should be used.

C. Which Babies Are At Risk for Polycythemia?

1. Babies who experience chronically low in utero oxygen levels

    Fetuses who were exposed to somewhat lower oxygen levels over a relatively long period will increase the number of red cells they produce to help improve their oxygenation. These include

    - Small for gestational age babies
    - Post-term babies

2. Babies who received extra blood from the placenta

    - *In utero twin-twin transfusion*: resulting from an abnormal connection between the placentas of twins; generally, the donor twin will be anemic while the recipient twin will be polycythemic
    - *In utero maternal-fetal transfusion*: resulting from abnormal connection(s) within the placenta causing the fetus to receive blood directly from the mother
    - *Delayed cord clamping* at the time of delivery

3. Babies who are large for gestational age, especially infants of diabetic mothers may be polycythemic. The reasons for this are not entirely clear.

4. Babies with certain chromosomal abnormalities, such as Down syndrome.

D. Which Babies With Polycythemia Need to Be Treated?

Complications of untreated polycythemia may include thromboembolic events such as cerebral artery thrombosis, necrotizing enterocolitis, and acute tubular necrosis. Long-term motor and mental disabilities have also been associated with untreated polycythemia.

Currently there is some controversy over which babies should be treated. In general, however, most experts agree that the following babies need treatment:

- Babies with venous or arterial hematocrits greater than or equal to 70%
- Babies with venous or arterial hematocrits between 65% to 70% who have signs or symptoms of polycythemia

3. How Is a Reduction Exchange Transfusion Done?

The procedure for performing a reduction exchange transfusion is similar to an exchange transfusion done for hyperbilirubinemia. The difference is blood is withdrawn from the baby and saline is given to the baby instead of blood.

The purpose of a reduction exchange transfusion is to reduce the baby's red cell mass. Therefore, some of the thick (polycythemic) blood is removed and a solution that will dilute the baby's blood is infused. In addition, a full exchange is not performed. Only enough blood to lower the baby's hematocrit to an acceptable range is exchanged.

A. How Do You Calculate the Amount of Blood to Exchange?

Use the formula given below to determine the amount of blood that should be withdrawn from a baby. The amount of blood withdrawn is also the amount of diluent (normal saline) that should be given to the baby.

Blood to Withdraw

$$\text{baby's blood volume} \times \frac{\text{actual Hct} - \text{desired Hct}}{\text{actual Hct}} = \text{amount of blood to withdraw}$$

(Hct = hematocrit)

Normal Saline to Infuse

calculated amount of blood to be withrawn = amount of saline to infuse

Example: A 3,000-g (6 lb, 10 oz) baby has a hematocrit of 75%. The baby's blood volume is 90 mL/kg (Book II: Neonatal Care, Blood Pressure). The baby's total blood volume, therefore, is 270 mL (90 mL × 3 kg = 270 mL). You wish to reduce the hematocrit to 55%.

$$270\ \text{mL} \times \frac{75\% - 55\%}{75\%}$$

$$270\ \text{mL} \times \frac{20}{75}$$

270 mL × 0.26 = 70 mL of blood to withdraw from the baby and
70 mL of normal saline to infuse

B. What Methods Are Used to Perform a Reduction Exchange Transfusion?

- **Pull-push technique:** 5 to 10 mL of the baby's blood is withdrawn (pulled) through a UVC and discarded, followed by normal saline infused (pushed) through the UVC. This pull-push cycle is repeated until the desired volume of blood has been exchanged (see calculation above).

- **Continuous method:** withdrawal of blood from one line and simultaneous infusion of normal saline through a second line.

Blood may be withdrawn through a UAC, UVC, or PAC. Saline may be given through a PIV line or a UVC, if the tip of the catheter is in the inferior vena cava. Some experts consider the preferred routes are withdrawal through a PAC and replacement infusion through a PIV line.

Withdrawal of blood and infusion of normal saline need to be done *slowly* to avoid sudden shifts in the baby's blood pressure. Sudden shifts in blood pressure have been associated with intraventricular bleeding in newborns, particularly in preterm infants.

Withdrawal rate no faster than 2 to 3 mL/kg/minute and infusion rate no faster than 2 to 3 mL/kg/minute is recommended.

4. What Are the Potential Complications of a Reduction Exchange Transfusion?

Complications of a reduction exchange transfusion are similar to those outlined earlier for exchange transfusions for hyperbilirubinemia, but do *not* include complications directly related to use of whole blood products. For example, the risk of viral infections associated with the transfusion of blood is not a possible complication of a reduction exchange transfusion because blood is not given to the baby.

Some experts suggest waiting to feed an infant for 24 to 72 hours after a reduction exchange transfusion. Polycythemia by itself is associated with intestinal injury and necrotizing enterocolitis.

Self-Test

Now answer these questions to test yourself on the information in the last section.

C1. **True** **False** Untreated polycythemia has been associated with permanent mental disability.

C2. Blood for determining a baby's hematocrit should be taken from _____.

C3. List at least 5 possible signs of polycythemia.

_____

_____

_____

_____

_____

C4. In general, babies with hematocrit values equal to or greater than _____ % need to be treated for their polycythemia.

C5. A 1,980-g (4 lb, 6 oz) 38-week baby that is small for gestational age is tachypneic with a hematocrit of 66%. You rule out other causes for her respiratory distress and determine she needs a reduction exchange transfusion. How much blood would you exchange if her desired hematocrit is 50%?

_____ mL blood withdrawn

_____ mL normal saline given

Check your answers with the list near the end of the unit, immediately before the posttest. Correct any incorrect answers and review the appropriate section in the unit.

Direct Blood Transfusions in the Management of At-Risk and Sick Infants

1. What Is a Direct Transfusion?

A direct transfusion is the process of infusing packed red blood cells into a baby through a PIV line.

2. Why Are Direct Transfusions Done?

Direct transfusions are done to

- Replace blood previously withdrawn for laboratory studies.

- Maintain relatively high hematocrit levels in sick babies with respiratory distress to maintain or improve the oxygen-carrying capacity of the baby's blood.

- Treat babies who are hypovolemic.

- Treat babies who have signs of anemia.

3. Which Babies Need to Be Treated With Direct Transfusions?

 Because a very small risk of infection (HIV, hepatitis, etc) from blood transfusion still exists, as few transfusions as possible are performed. However, some babies will require at least one, or perhaps many, transfusions.

A. Babies Who Have Blood Taken for Laboratory Studies

Often sick or at-risk babies have numerous laboratory studies, which cumulatively result in a large quantity of blood being withdrawn. In general, in a sick baby who is requiring assisted ventilation, packed red cells are given when 10% of the baby's blood volume has been withdrawn over a relatively short period (eg, 2–3 days).

Example: A 1,000-g baby has a blood volume of 90 mL (90 mL/kg), therefore, when 10% x 90 mL or 9 mL of blood has been withdrawn from the baby in fewer than 3 days, many experts recommend a replacement transfusion of 9 mL of packed red blood cells.

If a baby is only mildly ill and has stable vital signs, you may decide to withdraw more than 10% of the baby's blood volume before replacing it.

B. Sick Babies Who Require Ventilatory Support

Some babies who are very sick and require ventilatory support for respiratory, cardiac, or infectious problems are transfused to improve the oxygen-carrying capacity provided by their red blood cells. Many experts advise transfusing such babies to maintain their hematocrits at 40% or higher. Sick babies may need transfusions to maintain a hematocrit of 40%, even if very little blood has been withdrawn for laboratory studies.

C. Babies Who Are Hypovolemic

Babies who are, or are suspected of being, hypovolemic due to blood loss may be given direct transfusions to increase their blood volume. The management of babies with hypovolemia is discussed in greater detail in Book I, Resuscitation and Book II: Neonatal Care, Blood Pressure.

D. Babies Who Have Signs of Anemia

Normally, even without any blood being withdrawn for laboratory studies, healthy term babies will become anemic during the first 6 to 8 weeks after birth. Preterm babies, or babies who have had blood withdrawn for laboratory studies, usually develop anemia sooner, and with a greater drop in hematocrit, than healthy term babies. Stable preterm babies often continue to grow well and have normal vital signs, even though they may become quite anemic with hematocrit levels of 25% or lower.

Some anemic babies, however, will demonstrate signs of anemia that may require a direct transfusion(s) to resolve the problems. Signs of anemia include

- Tachycardia
- Tachypnea
- Apnea
- Failure to gain weight

The decision of when to transfuse a baby who is anemic is controversial. Most experts recommend *not* transfusing babies who are anemic but have no signs or symptoms of anemia. When a baby develops signs such as tachycardia, tachypnea, or apnea, you should evaluate the baby for all the possible causes of these problems (Book III, Unit 1, Vital Signs and Observations).

If the most likely cause of the baby's problems is anemia, you need to weigh the risks of transfusion against the risks of the problems the baby is demonstrating. When signs of anemia are significant, and the baby's hospitalization is being prolonged because of these problems, a transfusion of packed red blood cells may be necessary.

4. How Is a Direct Transfusion Done?

- Packed red blood cells should be compatible with the baby's blood.
- Usually a volume of 10 to 15 mL/kg is transfused.

Example: A sick 1,500-g preterm infant requiring ventilator support has a hematocrit of 38%. You elect to transfuse the baby with 10 mL/kg.

10 mL × 1.5 kg = 15 mL of packed red cells to be transfused

- Packed red cells are given through a PIV line.

- Follow your hospital's protocol for acquiring parental consent and for the filtering, identification, and disposal of blood.

- A transfusion is usually given over approximately 3 to 4 hours. A transfusion that is given too quickly may cause volume overload, which may lead to increased respiratory distress in the baby.

- In a sick baby, the hematocrit should be checked 12 to 24 hours after transfusion. This allows time for the transfused blood to equilibrate in the baby's circulation. In a stable baby, you can generally wait to check the hematocrit until the next time blood is drawn.

5. What Are the Potential Complications of a Direct Transfusion?

A. Infection

Serious infections such as HIV or hepatitis can occur after blood transfusion. Currently blood banks extensively test blood before it is used. Despite these efforts, a very small number of individuals receiving blood may develop an infection.

B. Emboli

Small blood clots can pass through an IV line. Blood is usually filtered by the blood bank before it is sent to the nursery. If this is not done, a filter should be inserted between the blood being transfused and the baby before the transfusion is given.

C. Elevated Potassium Levels

Older blood can have high levels of potassium. In general this is not dangerous because the total amount of potassium that will be given to the baby is small; however, in very small, sick babies an added potassium load can result in an elevation of potassium to a level that can cause heart arrhythmias. Therefore, you should always use the freshest blood available.

Self-Test

Now answer these questions to test yourself on the information in the last section.

D1. **True** **False** Some babies will require a transfusion of packed red blood cells when their hematocrits fall below 40%, while other babies with hematocrits of 25% or lower will not require a transfusion.

D2. List 4 reasons transfusions of packed red blood cells are used.

_____

_____

_____

_____

D3. **True** **False** Certain viral infections may occur as a result of a blood transfusion.

D4. Blood should be filtered before it is transfused to prevent the infusion of _____.

Check your answers with the list near the end of the unit, immediately before the posttest. Correct any incorrect answers and review the appropriate section in the unit.

Exchange, Reduction, and Direct Transfusions

Recommended Routines

All of the routines listed below are based on the principles of perinatal care presented in the unit you have just finished. They are recommended as part of routine perinatal care.

Read each routine carefully and decide whether it is standard operating procedure in your hospital. Check the appropriate blank next to each routine.

Procedure Standard in My Hospital	Needs Discussion by Our Staff	
_____	_____	1. Establish a policy of obtaining an x-ray for umbilical catheter placement before an exchange transfusion.
_____	_____	2. Establish a policy of providing continuous electronic cardiac monitoring for all babies undergoing an exchange transfusion.
_____	_____	3. Establish a policy of monitoring blood pressure at least every 15 minutes during an exchange transfusion.
_____	_____	4. Establish a routine of determining hematocrit, serum glucose, calcium, potassium, sodium, and bilirubin after every exchange transfusion.
_____	_____	5. Establish a routine of warming blood before an exchange transfusion, using a commercial blood warmer with appropriate temperature control and alarm features.
_____	_____	6. Establish a policy of using phototherapy after any exchange transfusion for hyperbilirubinemia.
_____	_____	7. Establish a policy of checking the hematocrits of all babies at risk for polycythemia.
_____	_____	8. Establish a policy of using only venous or arterial (not capillary) blood to determine the hematocrit of a newborn at risk for polycythemia.
_____	_____	9. Establish a policy of monitoring all babies with hematocrits greater than 65% for signs of polycythemia.
_____	_____	10. Establish a policy of recording and tallying the amount of blood withdrawn from a baby.
_____	_____	11. Establish a policy of monitoring the hematocrits of sick babies and stable, growing preterm babies.
_____	_____	12. Establish a policy of monitoring babies with low hematocrits for signs of anemia.

These are the answers to the self-test questions. Please check them with the answers you gave and review the information in the unit wherever necessary.

A1. Hypocalcemia
Hypoglycemia
Acidosis/alkalosis
Hyperkalemia

A2. 45% to 55%

A3. False   Blood should only be warmed with a commercial blood warmer that has the appropriate temperature control and alarm features.

A4. One third to one half

A5.

	Withdraw		Infuse	
	Yes	No	Yes	No
Umbilical arterial catheter	x	___	___	x
Peripheral arterial catheter	x	___	___	x
Umbilical venous catheter	x	___	x	___
Peripheral intravenous line	___	x	x	___

B1. False   Blood may be withdrawn from an artery but should not be infused into an artery. The risk of tissue damage from accidental infusion of air bubbles or tiny clots is much greater with an infusion through an artery than through a vein.

B2. Any 2 of the following:
- Arrhythmia
- Volume overload or depletion
- Cardiorespiratory arrest

B3. 4 to 6 hours

B4. Any 3 of the following:
- Hypocalcemia
- Hypoglycemia
- Hyperkalemia
- Hypernatremia
- Rebound hyperbilirubinemia

C1. True

C2. Artery or vein (*not* heel stick)

C3. Any 5 of the following:
- Plethora
- Cyanosis
- Lethargy
- Poor feeding
- Respiratory distress
- Congestive heart failure
- Tremors
- Seizures
- Hypoglycemia
- Hyperbilirubinemia

C4. 70%

C5. 44 mL blood withdrawn $180 \times \dfrac{66 - 50}{66} = 44\,\text{mL}$

    44 mL normal saline given

D1. True
D2. A. Replace blood withdrawn for lab tests.
     B. Treat hypovolemic babies.
     C. Treat stable babies who have symptomatic anemia.
     D. Maintain hematocrit level of approximately 40% in sick babies.
D3. True, although risk is extremely small.
D4. Tiny blood clots

Unit 4 Posttest

Without referring back to the information in the unit, please answer the following questions. Select the **one best** answer to each question (unless otherwise instructed). Record your answers on the answer sheet that is the last page in this book *and* on the test.

1. **True** **False** Treatment of hypocalcemia may be necessary during or shortly after an exchange transfusion.

2. **True** **False** Exchange transfusions should never be used for babies with bilirubin levels lower than 20 mg%.

3. **True** **False** An umbilical venous catheter may be used to withdraw and infuse blood during an exchange transfusion.

4. **True** **False** Packed red blood cells (hematocrit >70%) of appropriate group and type should be used for an exchange transfusion.

5. The tip of a venous catheter used to perform an exchange transfusion should be in the
   A. Left atrium of the heart
   B. Femoral vein
   C. Abdominal aorta
   D. Inferior vena cava

6. How should donor blood best be warmed?
   A. With a commercial blood warmer
   B. Under a radiant warmer
   C. In a warm water bath with the temperature set for 40°C (104°F)
   D. Under phototherapy lights

7. The hematocrit of donor blood used for an exchange transfusion should be between
   A. 30% to 40%
   B. 45% to 55%
   C. 60% to 70%
   D. 75% to 85%

8. Which of the following complications is *least* likely to be associated with an exchange transfusion for hyperbilirubinemia?
   A. Rebound hyperbilirubinemia
   B. Hypoglycemia
   C. Polycythemia
   D. Hypocalcemia

9. All of the following are possible signs of anemia *except*
   A. Apnea spells
   B. Hypothermia
   C. Tachypnea
   D. Tachycardia

10. Which of the following is recommended as replacement fluid in a reduction exchange transfusion?
    A. Lactated Ringer's solution
    B. Plasma protein fraction
    C. $D_{10}W$
    D. Normal saline

11. Direct transfusions of packed red blood cells are used for all of the following *except* to
    A. Treat infection.
    B. Replace blood drawn for laboratory tests.
    C. Treat hypovolemic shock.
    D. Treat severe anemia.

12. All of the following are possible signs of polycythemia *except*

   A. Seizures
   B. Respiratory distress
   C. Hyperglycemia
   D. Hyperbilirubinemia

13. True   False   All at-risk and sick babies should be transfused with packed red blood cells when their hematocrits drop below 40%.

14. True   False   A term baby who is small for gestational age and has a venous hematocrit of 72% but has no signs of polycythemia should receive a reduction exchange transfusion.

For each question, please make sure you have marked your answer on the test and on the answer sheet (last page in book). The test is for you; the answer sheet will need to be turned in for continuing education credit.

Skill Unit   Exchange Transfusions

This skill unit will teach you how an exchange transfusion is performed. Not everyone will be required to learn how to conduct an exchange transfusion; however, everyone should read this unit and attend a skill session to learn the equipment and sequence of steps so they can assist with the preparation for an exchange transfusion.

Although the mastery steps listed below are the same as the ones used in clinical practice to perform an exchange transfusion, manikins and models should be used for demonstration and practice of this skill.

The staff members who will be asked to master all aspects of this skill will need to demonstrate correctly each of the following steps:

1. Prepare the "baby" (manikin) for the exchange transfusion.

2. Prepare the donor "blood."

3. Insert an umbilical venous catheter, umbilical or peripheral arterial catheter, and/or peripheral intravenous line, as needed.

4. Demonstrate the pull-push method and/or the continuous method.

5. Record blood exchanged, vital signs, etc.

6. Monitor the "baby" during the exchange.

7. Monitor the "baby" after the exchange.

Performing Exchange Transfusions

Note: While this skill unit describes the procedure for an exchange transfusion for hyperbilirubinemia, the same basic techniques are used for a reduction exchange for polycythemia. As you know, the amount of blood withdrawn and the replacement fluid given are both different, but the techniques for how the blood is withdrawn and how the volume is replaced are the same.

Actions	Remarks

Preparing the Baby for an Exchange Transfusion

Several things must be done to prepare a baby before the actual exchange transfusion begins. These are

1. Send a sample of baby's and mother's blood for crossmatching.

2. Do not give enteral feedings (NPO) for 3 to 4 hours or aspirate stomach contents just prior to the exchange.

   Remark: This will reduce the chance the baby will vomit (and possibly aspirate) during the procedure.

3. Establish a properly warmed and oxygenated (if the baby requires supplemental oxygen) environment for the baby during the exchange.

   Remark: Exchange transfusions can be done with the baby inside an incubator or under a radiant warmer. Wherever care is provided, it must be possible to establish and maintain a sterile field.

4. Begin a peripheral intravenous (PIV) line.

   Note: If a PIV line is being used to infuse blood during a continuous exchange, a *second* PIV line will be needed to infuse routine IV fluids.

   Remark: During the exchange, the amount of blood given will usually be the exact amount withdrawn. A separate IV is needed to provide a constant infusion of fluid and glucose during the exchange, and to provide IV access in case of an emergency.

5. Attach a cardiac monitor to the baby. This monitor should provide a continuous signal of the baby's heartbeat. High and low heart rate alarms should be set.

   Remark: Continuous cardiac monitoring is important so any change in the baby's heart rate can be detected instantaneously.

6. Attach a blood pressure cuff to one of the baby's extremities and obtain a measurement at least every 15 minutes.

   Remark: Because the baby may get too much or too little volume during the procedure, or develop a complication, it is important to monitor blood pressure.

7. Collect resuscitation equipment and place it at the baby's bedside. This equipment includes

   - Resuscitation bag and mask (assembled and connected to an oxygen source)
   - Laryngoscope, endotracheal tubes, stethoscope, etc
   - Emergency medications
   - At least 2 people trained in neonatal resuscitation present with the baby throughout the entire procedure

   Remark: The mortality rate associated with exchange transfusions is less than 1%; however, unexpected, unexplained cardiac arrest does occur occasionally.

   Fewer and fewer perinatal health care providers are experienced with exchange transfusions. This makes being prepared for the unexpected increasingly important.

107

Actions	Remarks

Preparing the Baby for an Exchange Transfusion (continued)

8. Prepare the blood.

   a. Be sure the blood is antigen-negative for passively acquired antibodies.

   b. Know the anticoagulant used and the age of the blood. Request blood that is 10 days old or less.

   See 4 in Exchange Transfusions for Hyperbilirubinemia.

   For citrate phosphate dextrose adenine (CPDA-1) anticoagulated blood, be especially careful to observe the baby for signs of hypocalcemia, and check for the possible development of hypoglycemia.

   Donor blood, especially older blood, will need to be washed by the blood bank to reduce potassium levels.

   c. Calculate the volume of blood needed.

   Generally, 2-volume exchange transfusions using 180 mL of donor blood for every kilogram of the baby's weight are used.

   Example: 2-volume exchange transfusion for a baby weighing 2,600 g (5 lb, 12 oz) would require 468 mL of donor blood (180 mL/kg × 2.6 kg = 468 mL).

   d. Request the hematocrit of the blood be between 45% to 55%.

   Most blood banks can prepare donor blood so it has an appropriate hematocrit.

   Do *not* use true packed red blood cells with high hematocrit values. See 6A in Exchange Transfusions for Hyperbilirubinemia.

   e. Warm the blood to 37°C (98.6°F) by using a commercial blood warmer that has

   • Constant temperature readout

   • Adjustable thermostat

   • Automatic alarm system to prevent warming the blood above 38.0°C (100.4°F)

   Do *not* use blood warmers without precise thermostatic control because these may cause mechanical trauma to the red blood cells.

   Do *not* heat the blood under a radiant warmer or in a water bath warmer than 38°C (100.4°F) because this may "tan" the surface red blood cells and produce intravascular hemolysis.

9. Prepare the fluid lines.

   Use the sterile procedure and insertion technique outlined in Book II: Neonatal Care, Umbilical Catheters, skill unit.

   a. Insert an umbilical venous catheter (UVC) if you will use the pull-push method.

   • Measure the baby to determine the appropriate distance to insert the UVC.

   • Use a size 5F catheter for tiny babies, a size 8F catheter for most babies.

   Maintain sterile technique throughout the catheterization and exchange transfusion. All involved should wear sterile gowns and gloves. If the baby is inside an incubator, masks are not necessary but should be used if the baby is on a radiant warmer.

108

Actions	Remarks

Preparing the Baby for Exchange Transfusion (continued)

b. Insert an umbilical arterial catheter (UAC), peripheral arterial catheter (PAC), UVC and/or PIV line if you are using the continuous method.

See 7A in Exchange Transfusions for Hyperbilirubinemia.

If the baby does not require a UAC for other reasons (eg, monitoring arterial blood gases, blood pressure), either the pull-push method through the UVC or the continuous method through a UVC and a PIV line is preferable.

Some practitioners place a PAC and use it for withdrawal, with infusion through a UVC or PIV line.

10. Determine the placement of the catheter(s) by x-ray.

- Ideally, a UVC tip should be at the junction of the inferior vena cava and right atrium.

- On x-ray, the UVC tip should be above or at the level of the diaphragm (see illustration).

- It is also possible to perform an exchange transfusion through a UVC when the catheter tip is still in the umbilical vein and will not pass into the inferior vena cava. However, there is a somewhat greater risk of liver damage. In this case, the catheter should be inserted only 1 to 2 cm and infusion of sclerosing drugs, such as calcium, should be avoided.

Wherever the UVC is placed, you should be able to obtain blood flow into the catheter very easily.

- A UAC tip should be between L3 and L4. (UAC catheter is not shown in the illustration. See Book II: Neonatal Care, Umbilical Catheters.)

- A PAC is commonly placed in the radial artery.

11. Collect the appropriate equipment. Commercially available sterile exchange transfusion kits are available, or you can make your own kit with the following equipment:

Pull-push method

- One 4-way stopcock
- 6-, 10-, or 12-mL syringe

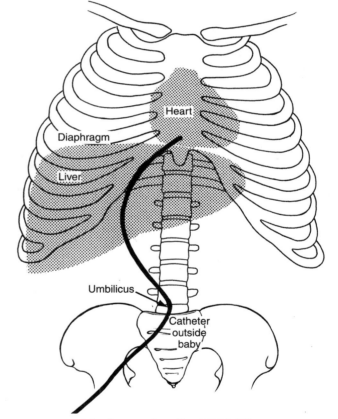

Ideal Location for UVC Tip

Actions	Remarks

Preparing the Baby for an Exchange Transfusion (continued)

Continuous method

- Three 3-way stopcocks
- One 50- to 60-mL syringe for each 150 mL of blood to be withdrawn
- One 50- to 60-mL syringe for blood infusion
- 5- to 6-mL syringe for heparinized saline flush

Either method

- Blood filter (sometimes blood filters are incorporated into IV tubing)
- IV tubing between the donor blood and stopcock
- Plastic bag or container to collect blood removed
- IV tubing between stopcock and collection container
- Two 5-mL syringes to obtain pre- and post-exchange laboratory samples

Performing an Exchange Transfusion

12. Assemble the equipment as shown in one of the diagrams that follow, depending on whether you will use the pull-push or continuous method.

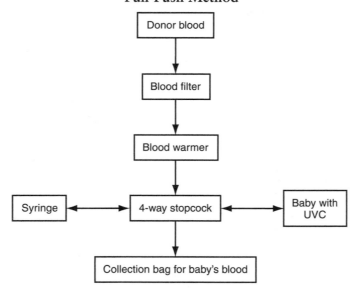

Pull-Push Method

110

Actions	**Remarks**

Performing an Exchange Transfusion (continued)

13A. *Pull-Push Technique*

  a. Open the UVC to the 10- or 12-mL syringe.

  b. Pull 5 or 10 mL of blood *slowly* from the baby, at a rate no faster than 2 to 3 mL/kg/minute.

  c. Turn the stopcock off to the UVC and open to the collection container.

  d. Push the blood out of the syringe and into the collection container.

  e. Turn the stopcock off to the collection container and open to the donor blood.

  f. Withdraw 5 or 10 mL (an amount equal to the volume just withdrawn from the baby) from the blood donor unit.

  g. Close the stopcock to the donor unit and open it to the UVC.

  h. *Slowly* push the donor blood out of the syringe and into the UVC, at a rate no faster than 2 to 3 mL/kg/minute.

  i. Leave the stopcock open to the UVC and *slowly* withdraw another 5 or 10 mL of blood from the baby.

Continue this pattern of pulling blood from the baby, discarding it, and pushing donor blood into the baby until 180 mL/kg of baby's weight of donor blood has been exchanged.

  j. It should take approximately 1 to 2 hours (depending on the amount of blood to be exchanged) to complete a pull-push exchange.

Remarks column:

See Step 13B for a description of the continuous method.

For small babies, only 5-mL volumes should be withdrawn or given at a time. For larger babies (>3,000 g) with stable vital signs, the individual exchange amounts may be 10 mL.

Be sure to hold the syringe upright so that any air bubbles in the syringe will not be pushed accidentally into the baby.

Withdraw and replace the blood in a slow and steady fashion. Rapid shifts in blood volume can be quite hazardous to a baby.

There is no advantage to rushing through an exchange transfusion because the rate of the exchange has little effect on the amount of bilirubin removed and, as noted earlier, rapid shifts in fluid volume can be harmful.

Actions	Remarks

Performing an Exchange Transfusion (continued)

Continuous Method

Infusion System

```
Donor blood
    │
    ▼
Blood filter
    │
    ▼
Blood warmer
    │
    ▼
50-mL  ◄──►  3-way
syringe      stopcock
              │
              ▼
          Baby with
          UVC or PIV
          line
```

Removal System

```
Baby with PAC,
UAC, or UVC
    │
    ▼
3-way          Collection
stopcock #1 ──► bag for
                baby's
                blood
    │
    ▼
Syringe with   3-way
heparinized ──► stopcock #2
saline
    │
    ▼
50-mL
syringe
```

13B. *Continuous Method*

Infusion steps and removal steps should be done simultaneously.

Infusion steps

a. Turn the stopcock so the 50- to 60-mL syringe is open to the donor blood.
b. Fill the syringe with 50 mL of donor blood.
c. Turn the stopcock off to the donor blood and open it to the UVC or PIV line being used for infusion.
d. Begin to infuse the donor blood at 2 to 3 mL/kg/minute.
e. Repeat steps a through d above until the desired volume (usually 180 mL/kg) of donor blood has been infused.

It is important that the rate of infusion and withdrawal of blood remain equal and constant so that shifts in the baby's blood volume do not occur.

Removal steps

a. Turn stopcocks 1 and 2 so the 50- to 60-mL syringe is open to the PAC, UAC, or UVC being used to withdraw the baby's blood.
b. Withdraw the baby's blood at a rate of 2 to 3 mL/kg/minute.
c. When 50 mL have been withdrawn, turn stopcock 1 off to the catheter and open to the collection bag.
d. Quickly eject the blood into the collection bag.
e. Turn stopcock 1 off to the collection bag and open to the catheter.
f. Repeat steps a through d above. Perform steps g through j after every 150 mL of baby's blood have been withdrawn.
g. Turn stopcock 1 off to the catheter and replace the 50-mL or 60-mL syringe with a new one.
h. Open stopcock 2 between the heparinized saline (5 units of heparin per 1 mL saline) syringe and the catheter.
i. Open stopcock 1 to the catheter.

Actions   **Remarks**

Performing an Exchange Transfusion (continued)

j. Gently flush the catheter with 1 to 2 mL of heparinized saline. Periodically changing the 50-mL or 60-mL syringe and flushing the catheter will help prevent clot formation.

k. Repeat steps a through j above until the desired volume (usually 180 mL/kg) of blood has been withdrawn.

14. Using either method, the first 5 or 10 mL of blood withdrawn from the baby should be used for pre-exchange laboratory studies.
    - Bilirubin
    - Hematocrit
    - Electrolytes
    - Calcium
    - Other (coagulation studies, chromosomes, or other tests that may be indicated for the infant undergoing the exchange)

15. Record each volume of blood withdrawn and infused on a tally sheet. Use a form similar to the one at the end of this unit.

    At the end of the exchange, the total amount of blood given should equal the total amount of blood withdrawn.

Every time one operator withdraws blood from or gives blood to the baby, he or she should call out the volume to another person who records it.

The recorder also maintains a running total of how much blood has been withdrawn and how much blood has been given.

16. Check and record the baby's vital signs at least every 15 minutes during the exchange.

17. Observe for signs of hypocalcemia, including
    - Jitteriness
    - Seizures
    - Apnea

    If any of these signs develop

    a. Flush the catheter with normal saline.

    b. Give 100 to 200 mg calcium gluconate per kilogram slowly through the UVC or PIV line. Use 5% (50 mg/mL) concentration (dilute 10% calcium gluconate with equal parts sterile water to make 5%).

    c. Stop the calcium infusion immediately if the baby's heart rate begins to slow.

    d. Flush the catheter with normal saline, then continue with the exchange transfusion.

Hypocalcemia is more likely to develop when CPDA-1 preserved blood is used rather than when heparinized blood is used.

There are risks associated with the administration of IV calcium, therefore, it probably should not be given unless signs of hypocalcemia actually develop.

Calcium injected rapidly, especially through a UVC, can cause cardiac arrest. Be sure the calcium and subsequent flush solution is given slowly.

113

Actions	Remarks

Performing an Exchange Transfusion (continued)

18. Mix the donor blood several times during the exchange.

This is to prevent settling of the donor blood, which would result in the baby receiving mostly plasma at the end of the exchange.

19. Obtain a blood sample for post-exchange laboratory studies
    - Glucose
    - Bilirubin
    - Hematocrit
    - Electrolytes
    - Calcium
    - Coagulation studies

Use the last blood withdrawn from the baby for these studies.

Note: Within 30 minutes after the exchange transfusion has been completed, the bilirubin level may rebound to a level approximating the pre-exchange level. This is due to equilibrium being established between extravascular and plasma bilirubin concentrations.

It is unlikely that the bilirubin level will continue to rise that rapidly; however, it is important to continue to check the bilirubin every 4 to 6 hours after an exchange transfusion.

A baby with hyperbilirubinemia severe enough to require one exchange transfusion may require several exchange transfusions.

20. Remove the catheter(s) unless another exchange is anticipated. If a PIV line was used for blood infusion, it may be converted into an IV lock until needed.

Babies with evidence of severe hemolysis (eg, a baby who requires an exchange transfusion within the first few hours after birth) probably will require several exchanges. For these babies, leave the catheter(s) in place for several hours until the trend of bilirubin rise can be determined.

Caring for a Baby After an Exchange Transfusion

21. Continue to check the baby's vital signs every 15 to 30 minutes for 3 to 4 hours.

22. Monitor glucose hourly for several hours.

Hypoglycemia is more likely to occur after rather than during the exchange.

23. Reinstitute phototherapy.

Phototherapy should be used after every exchange transfusion.

24. Continue to observe for complications.

See 9 in Exchange Transfusions for Hyperbilirubinemia.

Date _____

Baby's name _____

Exchange transfusion # _____

Birth weight _____

Birth date _____ Time _____

Mother's blood group _____

Baby's blood group _____ Coombs _____

Blood used: group _____ Hct _____

Time exchange started _____

Time exchange ended _____

Staff conducting the exchange

_____

_____

_____

Laboratory values

Pre-exchange

Hematocrit _____ Potassium _____

Bilirubin _____ Sodium _____

Calcium _____ Chloride _____

Other _____

_____

Post-exchange

Hematocrit _____ Potassium _____

Bilirubin _____ Sodium _____

Calcium _____ Chloride _____

Glucose _____ Other _____

Coagulation studies _____

Total volume withdrawn
From baby _____

Total volume given
To baby _____

Time	Blood Out		Blood In		Temp / Env Temp	Pulse / Resp	BP / Bld Gluc Chk	Medication/Comments
	Amt	Total	Amt	Total				

Page # _____

Time	Blood Out		Blood In		Temp		Pulse		BP		Medication/Comments
	Amt	Total	Amt	Total		Env Temp		Resp		Bld Gluc Chk	

Unit 5

Continuous Positive Airway Pressure

Objectives

In this unit you will learn

A. How continuous positive airway pressure (CPAP) works

B. When CPAP should and should not be used

C. How CPAP is administered

D. When and how a baby is weaned from CPAP

Unit 5 Pretest

Before reading the unit, please answer the following questions. Select the *one best* answer to each question (unless otherwise instructed). Record your answers on the answer sheet that is the last page in this book *and* on the test.

1. Which of the following is an appropriate way to feed babies requiring continuous positive airway pressure (CPAP) for acute respiratory disease?

   A. Intravenous fluids
   B. Tube feedings
   C. Nipple feedings with a special nipple
   D. None of the above

2. For which of the following babies would CPAP be *most* appropriate?

   A. Post-term baby with choanal atresia
   B. Preterm baby who is cyanotic due to congenital heart disease
   C. Term baby with a pneumothorax
   D. Preterm baby with respiratory distress syndrome

3. **True   False**   All babies with respiratory disease should receive continuous positive airway pressure.

4. Which of the following best describes the purpose of CPAP?

   A. Control the baby's respiratory rate.
   B. Decrease the baby's metabolic rate.
   C. Increase the baby's arterial oxygen concentration.
   D. Decrease the baby's chance of developing a pneumothorax.

5. Which of the following indicates the general range of pressure used with nasal CPAP when used in the treatment of respiratory distress syndrome?

   A. 2 to 4 cm H_2O pressure
   B. 4 to 10 cm H_2O pressure
   C. 10 to 14 cm H_2O pressure
   D. 14 to 18 cm H_2O pressure

6. A baby with respiratory distress syndrome is receiving nasal CPAP at 8 cm H_2O pressure and an inspired oxygen concentration (FiO_2) of 60%. Arterial blood gas results at these settings reveal: PaO_2 = 94, $PaCO_2$ = 45, pH = 7.32. Which of the following is the *most* appropriate next step to take to adjust the baby's CPAP and oxygen therapy?

   A. Decrease the FiO_2 to 40%, decrease the nasal CPAP to 4 cm H_2O pressure.
   B. Decrease the FiO_2 to 50%, maintain the nasal CPAP at 8 cm H_2O pressure.
   C. Maintain the FiO_2 of 60%, discontinue the nasal CPAP.
   D. Maintain the FiO_2 of 60%, increase the nasal CPAP to 10 cm H_2O pressure.

For each question, please make sure you have marked your answer on the test and on the answer sheet (last page in book). The test is for you; the answer sheet will need to be turned in for continuing education credit.

1. What Is Continuous Positive Airway Pressure (CPAP)?

When babies breathe normally, they pull air into their lungs by contracting their diaphragms, then exhale by allowing the air to flow passively out of their lungs against the atmospheric pressure in room air. CPAP is a technique that allows babies to exhale against pressure that is slightly higher than atmospheric pressure.

Delivery of CPAP requires the baby's airway to be connected to a system that can be pressurized. The most common method of connecting the airway to a CPAP system is through nasal prongs.

2. How Does CPAP Work?

In lungs with normal compliance, alveoli stay open during expiration. In lungs with poor compliance (stiff lungs), alveoli tend to collapse during expiration. When this happens, the baby must re-expand the collapsed alveoli during each inspiration. Babies with respiratory distress syndrome have poor lung compliance.

CPAP is *not* a form of mechanical ventilation. Air and oxygen are not forced into the lungs during inhalation. The baby must continue to breathe spontaneously.

The pressure provided with CPAP prevents alveoli from collapsing during expiration. The grunting heard in babies with respiratory distress syndrome who are not receiving CPAP is due to the baby's own effort to hold open the alveoli by exhaling against a partially closed glottis (upper airway).

Oxygen diffuses across the thin membranes of the alveoli into surrounding capillaries. The blood flow then carries the oxygen from the lung capillaries to the heart and then to blood vessels throughout the body.

Oxygen cannot enter collapsed alveoli and, therefore, cannot reach the capillaries surrounding those alveoli. CPAP improves arterial oxygenation by keeping alveoli open and thus allowing more places for oxygen to enter the bloodstream.

3. Which Conditions Benefit From CPAP?

CPAP is effective in the treatment of lung disease due to poor lung compliance. It is most commonly used for babies with respiratory distress syndrome.

 CPAP is not useful, and may even be harmful, for babies with normal lung compliance.

In general, CPAP should *not* be used for babies with respiratory distress due to factors such as birth asphyxia, most types of cyanotic congenital heart disease, airway obstruction, pneumothorax, etc.

A few babies with respiratory distress due to factors other than respiratory distress syndrome and some small preterm babies with apnea may also benefit from CPAP. Management of babies with these special conditions will not be discussed in this unit.

4. When Should a Baby Receive CPAP?

Continuous positive airway pressure is most useful to treat babies who have mild respiratory distress syndrome that is not severe enough to require endotracheal intubation and mechanical ventilation. CPAP is also useful for babies who were intubated for surfactant therapy, then extubated after surfactant was given. Before CPAP is used, the baby should have a chest x-ray compatible with respiratory distress syndrome and will usually have grunting and/or chest retractions too.

Preterm babies born at less than approximately 30 weeks' gestation almost always have poor lung compliance after birth. Some experts recommend giving CPAP to such babies, even before they exhibit signs of respiratory distress syndrome, to prevent alveolar collapse and avoid the need for surfactant therapy.

5. How Is CPAP Given?

The system for delivering CPAP may be a mechanical ventilator set to CPAP mode or a device that is made solely for delivery of CPAP. Several points are especially important to remember when setting up and maintaining a CPAP system.

A. Flow Rate

There should be a sufficient liter-per-minute flow rate through the tubing to prevent the baby from re-breathing his or her own exhaled air. As a general guideline, a combined air and oxygen liter-per-minute flow rate of 8 to 12 L/minute should be used. Use a flow rate at the lower end of that range for smaller babies and at the higher end for larger babies.

B. Pressure Regulation

The CPAP delivered to a baby is measured in centimeters of water (cm H_2O). The mechanical ventilator should be set on CPAP mode and pressure adjusted by turning the appropriate dial on the front of the ventilator. The pressure delivered to the baby then registers on the front of the ventilator.

Pressure adjustment should not be attempted until the nasal prongs are positioned properly on the baby (see skill unit).

C. Safety Pop-Off Valve

Mechanical ventilators and stand-alone CPAP devices have safety valves built in to prevent CPAP pressures from reaching dangerously high levels. With nasal CPAP, the baby's mouth also acts as a natural pop-off valve. It should *not* be taped shut.

Because babies generally will breathe only through their noses, pressure applied through the nasal prongs usually will not escape from the open mouth until a pressure of approximately 10 cm H_2O or greater is reached. This allows adequate CPAP to be delivered to the lungs, but reduces the chance of the baby inadvertently receiving too much pressure.

Set the high-pressure alarm on the CPAP delivery system approximately 2 cm H_2O above the set CPAP pressure.

D. Stomach Vent

Insert an 8F feeding tube into the baby's stomach through the mouth. Tape the tube in place and leave the end *open*.

When nasal prongs are used to deliver CPAP, the air/oxygen mixture is forced primarily into the lungs, but some of the flow may be diverted down the esophagus and into the stomach. The open feeding tube provides a vent so that the stomach does not become distended with gas.

E. Oxygen Concentration

CPAP is a delivery system for oxygen/air and pressure. The concentration of oxygen delivered through that system must still be regulated according to oxygen saturation and/or arterial blood gas values. In general, a baby should be started on CPAP with the same inspired oxygen concentration (FiO_2) that was being delivered to the baby's oxyhood.

If a baby receiving nasal CPAP is crying vigorously, room air (21% oxygen) may be inhaled through the mouth. Be sure the baby has been quiet for several minutes before the state of oxygenation is assessed with an arterial blood gas determination. If the baby continues to cry and breathe through the mouth, an oxyhood *plus* nasal CPAP may be helpful to maintain constant oxygenation.

F. Feedings

Babies receiving CPAP for acute respiratory distress generally should *not* be fed formula or milk, either by tube or nipple. Gastrointestinal motility is decreased in sick babies with respiratory disease. This means that a feeding is likely to stay in the stomach longer.

Because of this, a baby is much more likely to regurgitate some of the milk (or formula) and/or gastric juices and aspirate this fluid. Severe aspiration pneumonia could result. It is, of course, extremely important to maintain intravenous therapy for any baby receiving CPAP.

Some babies who have recovered from severe respiratory distress but still require CPAP can be tube fed.

6. How Much Pressure Is Used?

When nasal CPAP is used for respiratory distress syndrome, 4 to 6 cm H_2O is generally the appropriate starting pressure. Lower pressure than this is usually ineffective.

Sometimes the pressure may need to be increased to as much as 8 to 10 cm H_2O. Lower CPAP may be needed if the baby received surfactant. Make adjustments according to oximetry and arterial blood gas measurement results.

7. How Is a Baby Weaned From CPAP?

As the baby's respiratory disease improves, decrease the FiO_2 according to arterial blood gas and pulse oximetry values. When the baby requires approximately 35% FiO_2, begin decreasing the CPAP pressure in steps of 1 to 2 cm H_2O pressure at a time.

With continued improvement in the baby's condition, alternate between lowering the FiO_2 and lowering the CPAP pressure. Oxygenation should be assessed constantly by pulse oximetry and intermittently by arterial blood gas measurements obtained after any significant change in CPAP pressure or FiO_2. Discontinue CPAP when the pressure has been lowered to 2 to 4 cm H_2O and blood gases are normal.

Continue the baby's oxygen therapy using an oxyhood. Be prepared to increase the FiO_2 slightly for a short while after CPAP is stopped. Adjust the FiO_2 according to oximetry and arterial blood oxygen levels.

Unit 5 Posttest

Without referring back to the information in the unit, please answer the following questions. Select the **one best** answer to each question (unless otherwise instructed). Record your answers on the answer sheet that is the last page in this book *and* on the test.

1. **True   False**   When nasal CPAP is used, an orogastric tube should be inserted through the baby's mouth into the stomach and left uncapped.

2. **True   False**   When CPAP is used for acute respiratory disease, babies are best fed by tube feedings.

3. Which of the following *best* describes the purpose of CPAP?

   A. Decrease the baby's metabolic rate.
   B. Prevent pneumonia.
   C. Control the baby's respiratory rate.
   D. Prevent alveoli from collapsing during expiration.

4. Which of the following is the *most* appropriate combined air and oxygen flow rate for nasal CPAP?

   A. 2 to 4 L/minute
   B. 4 to 8 L/minute
   C. 8 to 12 L/minute
   D. 12 to 16 L/minute

5. A baby with respiratory distress syndrome is receiving nasal CPAP at 8 cm H_2O pressure and an inspired oxygen concentration (FiO_2) of 40%. Arterial blood gas results at these settings reveal: $PaO_2 = 40$, $PaCO_2 = 36$, pH = 7.38. Which of the following is the *most* appropriate way to respond to these blood gas values?

   A. Maintain the FiO_2 of 40%, discontinue the CPAP.
   B. Increase the FiO_2 to 50%, maintain the CPAP at 8 cm H_2O pressure.
   C. Maintain the FiO_2 of 40%, increase the CPAP to 12 cm H_2O pressure.
   D. Decrease the FiO_2 to 30%, maintain the CPAP at 8 cm H_2O pressure.

6. If CPAP is set at 6 cm H_2O, which of the following is the *most* appropriate setting for the high-pressure alarm?

   A.   4 cm H_2O pressure
   B.   6 cm H_2O pressure
   C.   8 cm H_2O pressure
   D. 10 cm H_2O pressure

For each question, please make sure you have marked your answer on the test and on the answer sheet (last page in book). The test is for you; the answer sheet will need to be turned in for continuing education credit

Skill Unit

Delivery of Continuous Positive Airway Pressure

This skill unit will teach you how to set up and maintain a system for delivery of continuous positive airway pressure (CPAP) using nasal prongs. Not everyone will be required to learn how to administer CPAP. However, everyone should read this skill unit to learn the equipment and sequence of steps so they can assist with this treatment.

The staff members who will be asked to master all aspects of this skill will need to demonstrate correctly each of the following steps:

1. Collect and assemble equipment.

2. Establish desired oxygen concentration and flow rate in the CPAP system.

3. Select prong size; position and secure nasal prongs.

4. Insert orogastric tube; tape in place and leave open.

5. Regulate CPAP pressure.

6. Set high-pressure alarm.

Using Continuous Positive Airway Pressure

Actions   **Remarks**

Preparing the Equipment for Nasal CPAP Delivery

1. Collect the following equipment:

    - Nasal prongs
    - Material to secure the nasal prongs
    - Oxygen source
    - Air source
    - Mechanical ventilator with CPAP mode or stand-alone CPAP device
    - Heater/humidifier
    - In-line thermometer
    - Frame to support the tubing, if needed
    - Orogastric tube

2. Assemble all of the above equipment.

3. Make the following preparations for providing oxygen and positioning and securing the prongs:

    - Select the appropriate-sized nasal prongs.

      - *Extra small size* for babies weighing less than approximately 1,000 g (2 lb, 3 oz)

      - *Small size* for babies weighing between approximately 1,000 g and 1,500 g (2 lb, 3 oz–3 lb, 5 oz)

      - *Large size* for babies weighing more than approximately 1,500 g (3 lb, 5 oz)

        Note: Different brands of prongs may vary slightly in shape.

Position the assembled equipment next to the baby.

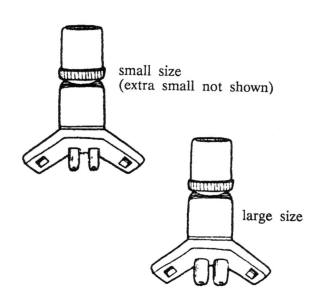

small size
(extra small not shown)

large size

Actions	**Remarks**

Preparing the Equipment for Nasal CPAP Delivery (continued)

• Coat prongs with a water-based lubricant.	With a cotton swab, dab a small amount of the lubricating cream on the prongs.
• Check the oxygen concentration flowing through the system.	
• Check the temperature registered on the in-line thermometer.	Be sure this is within the baby's neutral thermal environment (NTE) temperature range.
• Adjust the CPAP system flow rate.	Usually 8 to 12 L/minute flow is adequate.
• Occlude the tubing that connects to the prongs and check to see that the pressure reads zero.	Any pressure in the system will be delivered directly to the baby's lungs as soon as the tubing is connected to the nasal prongs. If this pressure is too high it could cause a pneumothorax.

Preparing the Baby for Nasal CPAP

• Methods to secure the nasal prongs.

a. Use a commercially available surgical mask that has one string on each of the 4 corners. Place this mask over the back of the baby's head. Use the strings to tie the nasal prongs in place.

When positioned correctly, the upper segment of the nosepiece should be vertical and at a right angle to the baby's face. The prongs should rest comfortably within the baby's nose.

Be careful to position the mask over the baby's occiput. It should *not* go over the back of the baby's neck or it will pull the nasal device in the wrong direction.

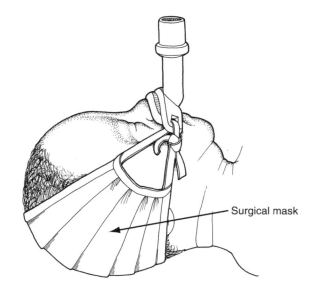

Surgical mask

OR
(see next page)

Actions	Remarks

Preparing the Baby for Nasal CPAP (continued)

b. Use Velcro and Stomahesive to secure the prongs.

    • Collect
       – Velcro
       – Stomahesive

    • Cut 2 circles from the Stomahesive, each approximately 3/4-inch in diameter, and 2 circles of slightly smaller diameter from the fish-hook side of the Velcro.

    • Stick the Velcro circles to the Stomahesive circles.

    • Cut an 8-inch strip of the softer fabric half of the Velcro.

    • Cut a slit in the center of this 8-inch fabric piece.

    • After slipping the upper segment of the nasal prongs through the slit, thread the free ends of the fabric through the openings in the flanges of the nasal prongs.

Remarks column:

Fish-hook side of the Velcro should have adhesive backing; fabric side should not.

Adjust size according to baby's size.

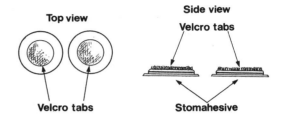

The slit should be approximately 1-inch long, just large enough to fit over the upper segment of the nasal prongs.

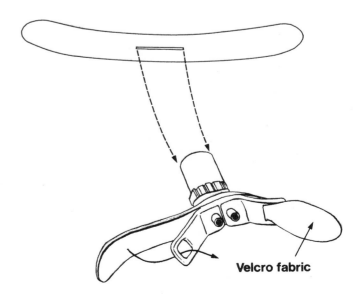

Actions	**Remarks**

Preparing the Baby for Nasal CPAP (continued)

- Place the Stomahesive tabs with the Velcro circles on the arches of the baby's cheekbones, directly in front of the ears.

- Position the nasal prongs in the baby's nose and attach the fabric ends of the Velcro to the fish-hook circles on the Stomahesive.

The upper segment of the nosepiece should be at a right angle to the baby's face.

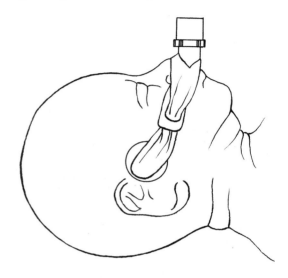

OR

c. Use commercially available prongs that are packaged with an apparatus designed to secure them.

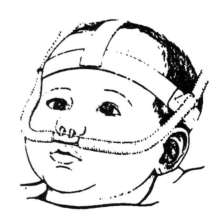

4. Position the prongs in the baby's nose and place the tubing in a neutral position so it does not pull or press against the baby's nose.

    The prongs should fit fully inside the baby's nostrils, but not press on the baby's nose or upper lip.

Actions	**Remarks**

Preparing the Baby for Nasal CPAP (continued)

5. Position the tubing

    • *If the tubing is suspended above the baby,* make rolls of cloth to place on either side of the baby's head.

    This will help steady the baby's head and keep the prongs in proper alignment. Babies may fuss initially, but if their heads are steadied for a few minutes and the prongs positioned properly, they will settle down and begin to breathe more comfortably.

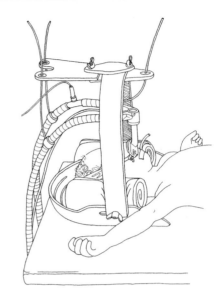

    • *If the baby's head is turned to one side,* a frame may not be needed to support the tubing.

Be sure that the

    • Upper segment of the nosepiece is at a right angle with the baby's face.

    • Tubing is taped securely to the bed so that it does not pull or press against the baby's nose.

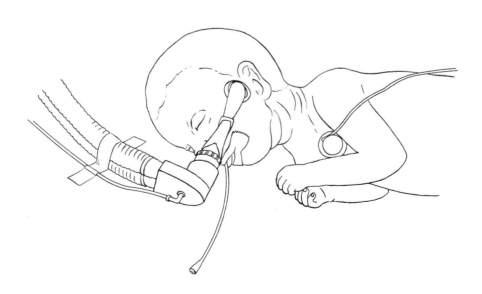

Actions	Remarks

Preparing the Baby for Nasal CPAP (continued)

6. Insert an orogastric tube, check its position, tape it in place, and leave it *open* to air.

    • This is a feeding tube that is inserted through the baby's mouth instead of the baby's nose.

    • Check the position of the tube by listening with a stethoscope over the stomach and injecting a small amount of air through the tube.

The purpose of the tube is to act as a vent, so the baby's stomach does not become distended from swallowed air. It is important, therefore, to leave the tube uncapped and periodically check for gastric distention.

Adjusting CPAP

7. Regulate the pressure by adjusting the CPAP pressure or positive end expiratory pressure (PEEP) knob on the ventilator or delivery device.

    • Generally pressures of 4 to 6 cm H_2O are used initially.

    • Lower or raise the pressure in 1 to 2 cm H_2O increments as the baby's condition indicates (as determined by arterial blood gases [ABGs] and oximetry).

    • Remove the CPAP apparatus and use an oxyhood to deliver the desired concentration of oxygen once the baby requires less than approximately 35% oxygen and 2 to 4 cm H_2O pressure.

8. Set the high-pressure alarm on the ventilator or CPAP delivery mechanism to signal if the pressure within the system reaches 2 cm H_2O above the set CPAP pressure.

In the illustration below, this knob is labeled "end-exp" for end expiratory pressure.

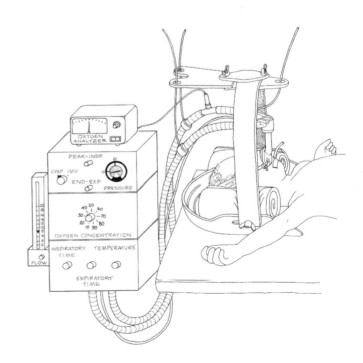

Actions	Remarks

Maintaining Nasal CPAP

9. Periodically check	For all of the items listed, check, record, and readjust, if necessary, at least once every hour.
• In-line temperature	Keep this within the baby's NTE range.
• Oxygen concentration	Whenever a baby receives oxygen therapy with an oxyhood, nasal CPAP, or endotracheal tube and mechanical respirator, it is essential to adjust the inspired oxygen concentration (FiO_2) according to oximetry and ABG results, and to monitor carefully the FiO_2 so sudden changes do not occur.
• CPAP pressure	Adjust this when the baby is quiet (not crying). Frequent readjustments may be necessary.
• Flow rate	Flow rate of 8 to 12 L/minute is generally adequate.
• Alignment of nosepiece	Adjust this according to the specific way in which the prongs you are using are designed to fit in relation to the baby's nose.

Unit 6

Assisted Ventilation With Mechanical Ventilators

Objectives

In this unit you will learn

A.   The principles of mechanical ventilation

B.   Which babies may require mechanical ventilation

C.   What criteria are used for starting mechanical ventilation

D.   How to set up a ventilator for babies with various types of respiratory problems

E.   How to adjust ventilator settings

 This unit is intended to teach only indications for and initiation of mechanical ventilation. It will not address long-term management of ventilated babies or weaning of babies from ventilators. Babies requiring mechanical ventilation should be managed in intensive care nurseries, where different philosophies about ventilator management may be practiced.

Unit 6 Pretest

Before reading the unit, please answer the following questions. Select the *one best* answer to each question (unless otherwise instructed). Record your answers on the answer sheet that is the last page in this book *and* on the test.

1. Which of the following can*not* be adjusted independently on most infant ventilators?

   A. Peak airway pressure
   B. End expiratory pressure
   C. Inspiratory time
   D. Inspired oxygen concentration
   E. Expiratory resistance

2. Which of the following is *least* reliable for determining the need for mechanical ventilation?

   A. Venous PCO_2
   B. Venous PO_2
   C. Arterial pH
   D. Arterial PCO_2
   E. Arterial PO_2

3. Which of the following is correct when determining ventilator settings for a baby with respiratory distress syndrome compared to a baby with normal lungs?

   A. End expiratory pressure should be higher.
   B. Inspiratory time should be shorter.
   C. Expiratory time should be longer.
   D. Peak inspiratory pressure should be lower.

4. In which of the following cases is mechanical ventilation *most* indicated?

   A. A 3,500-g (7 lb, 12 oz) baby with congenital pneumonia who is breathing 50% oxygen and has a PaO_2 of 60, $PaCO_2$ of 50, and a pH of 7.28.
   B. A 1,500-g (3 lb, 5 oz) baby with respiratory distress syndrome who is breathing 80% oxygen and has a PaO_2 of 45, $PaCO_2$ of 65, and a pH of 7.28.
   C. A 1,000-g (2 lb, 3 oz) baby with no lung disease who has an apneic spell that responds to tactile stimulation.
   D. A 3,000-g (6 lb, 10 oz) baby who had severe perinatal compromise and has a PaO_2 of 70, $PaCO_2$ of 25, pH of 7.20 while breathing 21% oxygen.

5. Which of the following is correct when determining ventilator settings for a term baby with meconium aspiration compared with a preterm baby with respiratory distress syndrome?

   A. Inspiratory time should be longer.
   B. Expiratory time should be shorter.
   C. End expiratory pressure should be higher.
   D. Rate should be faster.

6. Which of the following is *least* likely to suggest a blocked endotracheal tube?

   A. Poor chest movement
   B. High $PaCO_2$
   C. High pH
   D. Low PaO_2

For each question, please make sure you have marked your answer on the test and on the answer sheet (last page in book). The test is for you; the answer sheet will need to be turned in for continuing education credit.

1. What Is Mechanical Ventilation?

Mechanical ventilation assists, and sometimes controls, the breathing of babies who cannot move enough air with spontaneous respiration. An oxygen hood increases the concentration of oxygen a baby breathes. Continuous positive airway pressure (CPAP) prevents the alveoli from collapsing during exhalation, but only a mechanical ventilator provides artificial ventilation. The baby must be intubated with an endotracheal tube for treatment with a mechanical ventilator.

Mechanical ventilators work by forcing a humidified oxygen/air gas mixture into an intubated baby's lungs at a preset flow, maximum pressure, and time (inspiration). At the end of the inspiration time, the flow is stopped automatically. The gas is allowed to escape passively from the lungs, endotracheal tube, and ventilator tubing into the environment for another preset time (expiration). By altering the inspiratory and expiratory time, you are able to adjust how fast the mechanical ventilator will breathe for the baby (respiratory rate).

2. Which Babies Need Mechanical Ventilation?

Mechanical ventilation is required for babies who cannot move enough gas in and out of their lungs to achieve adequate oxygenation of the blood and/or adequate removal of carbon dioxide from the blood. Most of these babies will be in respiratory distress (Book II: Neonatal Care, Respiratory Distress).

Babies may require mechanical ventilation because of primary lung disease, such as respiratory distress syndrome, or because of respiratory depression from generalized illness, a congenital malformation, birth injury, or extreme prematurity. Examples include babies with severe recurrent apnea, diaphragmatic paralysis from birth injury, or hypoventilation from sepsis, brain hemorrhage, or some other central nervous system insult. Extremely preterm babies have weak respiratory musculature and may need mechanical ventilation, even if they do not have significant lung disease.

3. When Do You Start Mechanical Ventilation?

Mechanical ventilation is initiated when a baby demonstrates respiratory failure. Respiratory failure is defined as inadequate spontaneous ventilation even though the baby may be making considerable respiratory efforts. Arterial blood gases are the principal way to decide when respiratory failure occurs. Any one of the following factors is an indication for mechanical ventilation:

A. Very High or Rapidly Rising $PaCO_2$ and Low pH

Normal babies will automatically increase their breathing when blood carbon dioxide ($PaCO_2$) levels begin to rise. The increased respiratory rate results in lowering $PaCO_2$ to normal. Therefore, if $PaCO_2$ is high, the baby is not moving enough air in and out of functional lung tissue.

As $PaCO_2$ rises, pH falls. Consider mechanical ventilation when

- $PaCO_2$ is consistently greater than 60 mm Hg.
- $PaCO_2$ is consistently greater than 55 mm Hg and pH is less than 7.25.

B. Low PaO_2 Despite Appropriate Oxygen and CPAP Therapy

If lung disease becomes severe enough, the baby's own respiratory efforts will not be sufficient to provide adequate oxygenation. Consider mechanical ventilation if

- PaO_2 is less than 50 mm Hg with baby breathing 70% to 80% inspired oxygen.

Some experts believe that a baby with worsening respiratory distress syndrome can be effectively treated by being intubated, given surfactant, then extubated, and nasal CPAP started.

C. Extremely Preterm Baby

Although it is controversial, some experts advise electively intubating and mechanically ventilating extremely preterm babies (<1,000 g birth weight) at birth, rather than waiting for them to develop respiratory failure. Early, elective intubation is done to avoid acidosis and other problems likely to develop with respiratory failure. These tiny babies will also be candidates for surfactant therapy.

Other experts, however, believe that mechanical ventilation can be avoided by early use of nasal CPAP.

D. Surfactant Therapy

Intubation is required for surfactant administration (Unit 7, Surfactant Therapy in this book). Many of these babies will require mechanical ventilation for a time after surfactant is given.

E. Absence of Breathing (Apnea)

If a baby has apneic spells requiring repeated stimulation or bag-and-mask assistance, mechanical ventilation may be required. Continuous monitoring of oxygen saturation can also be helpful.

4. What Kind of Mechanical Ventilator Should Be Used?

There are many different brands of mechanical ventilators available. Some deliver a specific volume of gas, whereas others deliver a specific gas flow and pressure for a specific time. This unit will discuss only the more common pressure/flow/time-regulated ventilators. Be sure your ventilator has the following qualities:

A. Designed for Infants

Ventilators designed for adults usually do not have the fine adjustment capabilities required for infants.

B. Infant Tubing Circuit

Babies' lungs require only small volumes of gas. If the tubing that connects the ventilator to the endotracheal tube contains a large volume of gas, this gas will be compressed with each ventilator "breath." This causes the size of the breath that enters the endotracheal tube to be far smaller than the infant-sized breath initially produced by the ventilator. Therefore, the tubing should contain a small volume (diameter <2 cm) and be non-distensible.

C. Heated Humidifier With Thermostat Control in the Circuit

D. Oxygen Concentration Adjustable From 21% to 100%

Self-Test

Now answer these questions to test yourself on the information in the last section.

A1. *Most* infant mechanical ventilators work by
   A. Delivering a preset volume into the lungs
   B. Delivering a preset pressure for a preset time

A2. List 3 examples of babies who may require mechanical ventilation because of poor respiratory muscle function.

_____

_____

_____

A3. Respiratory failure requiring mechanical ventilation is indicated by

High _____

Low _____

Low _____

A4. Infant tubing circuits should have the following characteristics:

_____

_____

A5. **True   False**   Respiratory failure refers only to babies who stop breathing completely.

A6. List 2 indications for mechanical ventilation other than respiratory failure or severe apnea.

_____

_____

Check your answers with the list at the end of this unit, before the posttest. Correct any incorrect answers and review the appropriate section in the unit.

5. How Do You Set Up a Mechanical Ventilator?

The objective of mechanical ventilation is simple: to move air and oxygen sufficiently to normalize arterial blood gases. The method of achieving this will depend on the type of disease being treated. The following ventilator settings will need to be adjusted:

- *Peak inspiratory pressure (PIP):* This is the maximum pressure that the ventilator reaches to force gas into the lungs. If the pressure is too low, gas movement will be inadequate; if too high, the lungs can be damaged and a pneumothorax can be created.

- *Positive end expiratory pressure (PEEP):* This is the pressure during expiration and is identical to CPAP. If the expiratory pressure is too low, the alveoli may collapse (in babies with poor lung compliance); if too high, expiration will be restricted and gas movement will be inadequate.

- *Inspiratory time (T_I):* This is the time during which the ventilator delivers its inflation pressure. If T_I is too short, the PIP will not reach the alveoli and gas movement will be inadequate; if T_I is too long, exhalation will be inadequate. Prolonged T_I will also restrict lung blood flow due to compression of lung blood vessels by distended alveoli.

- *Expiratory time (T_E):* This is the time during which the baby passively exhales. If T_E is too short, expiration will be insufficient and gas will be trapped in the lungs, possibly causing lung damage and a pneumothorax. With most ventilators T_E cannot be set independently but is determined by T_I and the rate. Expiratory time is calculated with the following formula:

$$T_E = (60/\text{rate}) - T_I$$

For example, a ventilator for a baby with respiratory distress syndrome is set for an inspiratory time of 0.6 seconds and a rate of 45.

$$T_E = (60/45) - 0.6$$

$$T_E = 1.3 - 0.6$$

$$T_E = 0.7 \text{ seconds}$$

- *Rate:* The rate or breaths per minute is determined by the lengths of T_E and T_I. Most ventilators have a separate knob that allows adjustment of the rate. This knob works by changing the length of T_E. Thus you set only T_I and rate. If rate is too low or very high, gas movement will be inadequate. If rate is slightly high, gas movement will be excessive and $PaCO_2$ will be too low.

- *Oxygen concentration (FiO_2):* This should be adjusted from 21% to 100% as determined by oxygen saturation and/or arterial blood gas values, as outlined in Book II: Neonatal Care, Oxygen.

- *Flow rate:* This is the speed at which the ventilator delivers a breath. If flow rate is too low, it may not be possible for the ventilator to reach the desired PIP; if too high, the lungs may be damaged. For most babies, regardless of illness, approximately 8 L/minute will be adequate. If very high PIP or very fast ventilator rates are required, a higher flow rate may be necessary. Many of the newer ventilators do not have a separate setting for flow rate, because the flow rate adjusts electronically depending on the ventilation pattern selected.

- *Mean airway pressure (MAP):* MAP is the average pressure in the airway throughout the respiratory cycle. It is a function of PIP, PEEP, T_I, rate, and flow rate settings. It is not independently adjustable but will change when any one of the other settings is increased or decreased. The MAP value is displayed on most infant ventilators.

Along with FiO_2, MAP is important in determining a baby's oxygenation. When any one of the settings that affect MAP is changed, one of the other settings should be adjusted to keep MAP constant to keep PaO_2 relatively constant. In addition to FiO_2, adjustments in MAP may also be used to achieve an acceptable PaO_2.

Ranges of Ventilator Settings Available on Most Infant Ventilators

Setting	Abbreviation	Range	Unit
Peak inspiratory pressure	PIP	0–60	cm H_2O
Positive end expiratory pressure	PEEP	0–10	cm H_2O
Inspiratory time	T_I	0.2–1.0	Seconds
Expiratory time*	T_E	>0.3	Seconds
Rate	—	0–150	Cycles/minute
Oxygen concentration	FiO_2	21–100	Percent
Flow rate	—	0–20	Liters/minute

*Not able to be set independently on most ventilators; calculated from T_I and the rate. Most experts advise not allowing the inspiratory time ever to exceed the expiratory time.

6. What Initial Settings Are Used?

If you decide that mechanical ventilation is indicated, you should first stabilize the baby by assisting ventilation with bag and endotracheal tube breathing. During this time, the endotracheal tube should be secured in place and the ventilator set up at the bedside.

Set the PIP, PEEP, T_I, rate, flow rate, and FiO_2 *before the baby is connected.* Test these settings by occluding the opening of the connector, which will later be attached to the baby's endotracheal tube. Finer adjustments will be required after the baby is connected to the ventilator.

If a manometer is included in your bag-breathing system (see Book I, Resuscitation, Bag-and-Mask Ventilation skill unit), the ventilator PIP and rate may be set to match the most effective bag ventilation; therefore, note the maximum pressure and rate at which you are bag-breathing for the baby.

It is also important that you consider the disease process when deciding on initial settings. Relative settings for various conditions as well as specific initial settings are suggested on the next page.

Relative Ventilator Settings for Various Lung Conditions

- **Normal Lungs**
  (eg, apnea with no lung disease)

PIP	Low
PEEP	Low
T_I	Short
T_E	Long
Rate	Slow
FiO_2	Usually 21% (room air)

- **Airway Disease**
  (eg, meconium aspiration)

PIP	High
PEEP	Low
T_I	Short
T_E	Long
Rate	Fast
FiO_2	Equal to FiO_2 before mechanical ventilation

- **Alveolar Disease**
  (eg, respiratory distress syndrome or pneumonia)

PIP	High
PEEP	High
T_I	Long (but not longer than T_E)
T_E	Short
Rate	Slow
FiO_2	Equal to FiO_2 before mechanical ventilation

Suggested Initial Settings for Mechanical Ventilation

Disease State	PIP (cm H_2O)	PEEP (cm H_2O)	T_I (seconds)	Rate (per minute)	FiO_2 (%)	Flow* (L/min)
Alveolar (eg, respiratory distress syndrome, pneumonia)	25	4–5	0.4–0.6	40–60	†	8
Airway (eg, aspiration)	25	2–3	0.4	60	†	8
Normal Lungs (eg, apnea)	12	2	0.5	30	†	8

*Determined automatically by most newer ventilators.

†Individualize FiO_2 depending on FiO_2 before mechanical ventilation and results of pulse oximetry and/or arterial blood gas determinations.

Some babies will have a combination of problems and require settings between 2 categories. For example, a very tiny baby (<1,000 g) may have only mild respiratory distress syndrome but require mechanical ventilation because of very weak respiratory muscles. Although the baby has respiratory distress syndrome, much lower PIP and PEEP will probably be required than if the baby were bigger and/or had more severe lung disease. Many experts are advising short T_I and rapid rates to use lower PIP and perhaps cause less trauma to the lungs of very tiny babies.

7. How Do You Adjust a Ventilator After a Baby Has Been Connected?

After the ventilator has been connected to the baby, the PIP and PEEP may be slightly lower than you had set them earlier. This is expected because the baby's lungs have been added to the system. Before changing any settings, evaluate chest movement, skin color, oximetry, and blood gases.

The following chart suggests several possible actions for various abnormal findings. Which action you choose will depend on the initial settings of the ventilator, the disease you are treating, and the severity of disease.

Any ventilator change you make to correct one variable (such as PaO_2) is also likely to affect another variable (such as $PaCO_2$). Use continuous pulse oximetry and obtain an arterial blood gas approximately 10 to 30 minutes after any significant change in ventilator setting(s).

8. What Are Suggested Ventilator Adjustments for Various Clinical Findings?

 If the baby's condition changes, assess the baby and the functioning of the ventilator.

A. To Check the Ventilator, Consider
- Is the proper FiO_2 being delivered?
- Is the tubing loose or disconnected?
- Does the pressure reach the preset PIP with each breath?
- Does the pressure fall to the preset PEEP between each breath?
- Have the T_I, T_E, or rate settings been changed accidentally?

B. To Check the Baby, Consider

Chest movement	• **Rises and falls with each breath** – No change • **Moves little to not at all** – Check endotracheal tube placement – Check for blocked endotracheal tube (suction) – Increase PIP – Decrease PEEP – Increase T_I • **Moves too much** – Decrease PIP – Decrease T_I
Skin color	• **Pink and well-perfused** – No change

- **Blue**
  - Check endotracheal tube placement
  - Check for blocked endotracheal tube (suction)
  - If sudden cyanosis, check for pneumothorax
  - Increase FiO_2
  - Increase MAP*

- **Pale and mottled**
  - Decrease PEEP
  - Increase T_E
  - Consider non-respiratory etiology

Arterial blood gases	- PaO_2, $PaCO_2$, pH normal
	   - No change
	
	- PaO_2 low (<45 mm Hg)
	   - Check endotracheal tube placement
	   - Check for blocked endotracheal tube (suction)
	   - Increase FiO_2
	   - Increase MAP*
	
	- PaO_2 high (>75 mm Hg)
	   - Decrease FiO_2
	   - Decrease MAP*
	
	- $PaCO_2$ high (>55–60 mm Hg) and/or pH low (<7.25)
	   - Check endotracheal tube placement
	   - Check for blocked endotracheal tube (suction)
	   - If sudden change, check for pneumothorax
	   - Increase PIP
	   - Decrease PEEP
	   - Decrease T_I
	   - Increase rate
	
	- $PaCO_2$ low (<35 mm Hg) and/or pH high (>7.45)
	   - Decrease PIP
	   - Decrease rate

*If a ventilator adjustment is being made in response to an unacceptable $PaCO_2$, but with a normal PaO_2, keep the MAP constant by adjusting one of the other settings that also affects MAP. (See Section 5.) If the PaO_2 is too low or too high, adjust the FiO_2 first; then consider adjusting the MAP, usually by adjusting the PEEP or PIP.

9. What Can Go Wrong?

If requirement for mechanical ventilation is anticipated for longer than several hours, the baby should be transferred to an intensive care nursery.

 Mechanical ventilation of babies is an invasive, potentially dangerous therapy that requires constant attendance by an experienced team.

Possible complications

- *Air leaks:* Pneumothorax should be suspected immediately if the baby's condition suddenly deteriorates. Insertion of a chest tube may be life-saving. Air leaks into the lung tissue, pericardium, or mediastinum can also occur and are detectable by chest x-ray.

- *Blocked or displaced endotracheal tube:* If the endotracheal tube becomes dislodged from the trachea, or blocked with mucus, the ventilator will continue to cycle but the baby's vital signs will deteriorate. Suction the tube and attempt to ventilate the baby with a resuscitation bag connected to the endotracheal tube. Check breath sounds and chest movements. If there is no improvement in the baby's condition, remove the endotracheal tube and assist the baby's ventilation with bag and mask until a new endotracheal tube can be inserted.

- *Endotracheal tube slips in too far:* If the tube slips in too far, it may enter the airway of one lung and block air entry to the other lung. In this case, breath sounds will be unequal when you listen with a stethoscope over the right and left chest. Also one side of the chest may rise more than the other. If this occurs, pull the tube back slightly as you listen with a stethoscope for improved breath sounds.

- *Disconnected or malfunctioning ventilator:* Most ventilators are equipped with alarms that will sound if the tubing becomes disconnected. Even without an alarm, a tubing or power disconnect can be detected because the airway pressure gauge will not rise normally with each breath.

 If a ventilator malfunctions, don't panic! Simply connect a resuscitation bag to the endotracheal tube and bag-breathe the baby until the problem can be located and corrected.

10. What Else Should You Do for a Baby Receiving Mechanical Ventilation?

All babies receiving mechanical ventilation should have continuous electronic cardiac and pulse oximetry monitoring and experienced staff in constant attendance. Complete resuscitation equipment should be at the bedside.

Remember that continued monitoring for other risk factors (eg, hypoglycemia, hypothermia, etc) is essential to the baby's total care. These more routine activities should not get lost because a baby is receiving sophisticated respiratory support.

Self-Test

Now answer these questions to test yourself on the information in the last section.

B1. List 5 controls that require adjustment on most infant ventilators.

_____

_____

_____

_____

_____

B2. Circle the appropriate ventilator setting for each of the 3 lung conditions.

	Alveolar Disease	_Airway Disease_	_Normal Lungs_
Peak inspiratory pressure	High/Low	High/Low	High/Low
Positive end expiratory pressure	High/Low	High/Low	High/Low
Inspiratory time	Long/Short	Long/Short	Long/Short
Expiratory time	Long/Short	Long/Short	Long/Short
Rate	Slow/Fast	Slow/Fast	Slow/Fast

B3. List 3 observations or findings to consider before adjusting a ventilator.

_____

_____

_____

B4. List 4 common complications of mechanical ventilation.

_____

_____

_____

_____

Check your answers with the list on the next page. Correct any incorrect answers and review the appropriate section in the unit.

These are the answers to the self-test questions. Please check them with the answers you gave and review the information in the unit wherever necessary.

A1. B.   Delivering a preset pressure for a preset time.
A2. Any 3 of the following:
 • Severe generalized illness
 • Birth injury causing diaphragmatic paralysis
 • Hypoventilation from sepsis, brain hemorrhage, or some other central nervous system insult
 • Extreme prematurity
A3. High $PaCO_2$
 Low PaO_2
 Low pH
A4. Contain small volume of gas (tubing diameter <2 cm)
 Be non-distensible
A5. False   Babies who have inadequate ventilation despite spontaneous respirations are also in respiratory failure.
A6. Extreme prematurity (birth weight less than approximately 1,000 g)
 Surfactant therapy

B1. Peak inspiratory pressure
 Positive end expiratory pressure
 Inspiratory time
 Rate
 Oxygen concentration
B2.

	Alveolar Disease	*Airway Disease*	*Normal Lungs*
Peak inspiratory pressure	High	High	Low
Positive end expiratory pressure	High	Low	Low
Inspiratory time	Long	Short	Short
Expiratory time	Short	Long	Long
Rate	Slow	Fast	Slow

B3. Any 3 of the following:
 • Chest movement
 • Skin color
 • Breath sounds equal or unequal
 • Arterial blood gases
 • Percent oxygen saturation
B4. Air leaks, such as a pneumothorax
 Blocked or displaced endotracheal tube
 Endotracheal tube slips in too far
 Disconnected or malfunctioning ventilator

Unit 6 Posttest

Without referring back to the information in the unit, please answer the following questions. Select the **one best** answer to each question (unless otherwise instructed). Record your answers on the answer sheet that is the last page in this book *and* on the test.

1. If the inspiratory time is set at 1.0 seconds and the rate is set at 50, expiratory time will be

    A. Too long
    B. Too short
    C. Adequate

2. The tubing used for infant ventilators should

    A. Be easily distensible.
    B. Contain a small volume of gas.
    C. Be the same as used for adult ventilators.
    D. Have a large diameter.

3. Which of the following is a correct description of ventilator settings for a baby with respiratory distress syndrome compared to a baby with normal lungs?

    A. End expiratory pressure should be lower.
    B. Inspiratory time should be longer.
    C. Expiratory time should be longer.
    D. Peak inspiratory pressure should be lower.

4. Which of the following is a correct description of ventilator settings for a term baby with meconium aspiration compared to a preterm baby with respiratory distress syndrome?

    A. Inspiratory time should be longer.
    B. Expiratory time should be shorter.
    C. End expiratory pressure should be lower.
    D. Rate should be slower.

5. Which of the following is *most* likely to affect the ventilator rate?

    A. Flow rate
    B. Peak inspiratory pressure
    C. Expiratory time
    D. End expiratory pressure

6. A baby with respiratory distress syndrome is receiving mechanical ventilation and gradually develops hypoxemia (PaO_2 = 40 mm Hg). Which of the following ventilator settings is *least* likely to be the cause of the low PaO_2?

    A. Inspiratory time is too short.
    B. End expiratory pressure is too high.
    C. Peak airway pressure is too low.
    D. FiO_2 is too low.

For each question, please make sure you have marked your answer on the test and on the answer sheet (last page in book). The test is for you; the answer sheet will need to be turned in for continuing education credit.

Skill Unit

Endotracheal Tubes

This skill unit will teach you how to secure an endotracheal tube and how to suction an endotracheal tube. *Both of the skills described in this unit are to be carried out by teams of 2.*

Not everyone will be required to learn and practice these skills; however, everyone should read this unit and attend a skill session to learn the equipment and sequence of steps so they can assist with these skills.

The staff members who will be asked to master all aspects of this skill will need to demonstrate correctly each of the following steps:

Securing an Endotracheal Tube

Suture and Tape Method

1. Cut an Elastoplast "mustache."
2. Hold the endotracheal tube at the proper level.
3. Tape clear adhesive dressing and the Elastoplast to the "baby" (manikin).
4. Tie the endotracheal tube in place.
5. Tape the endotracheal tube in place with adhesive tape.
6. Listen to the "baby" to recheck correct tube placement.

Commercial Stabilizer Method

1. Select the appropriate-sized stabilizer for the tube.
2. Hold the endotracheal tube at the proper level.
3. Stick the stabilizer to the face on one side of the mouth.
4. Slide the tube into the stabilizer and lock in place.
5. Listen to the "baby" to recheck correct tube placement.

Suctioning an Endotracheal Tube

1. Collect the appropriate equipment and suction catheters for the tube and "baby" to be suctioned.
2. Adjust the suction pressure.
3. Determine the length of suction catheter to be inserted.
4. Bag-breathe for the "baby" using the appropriate pressure and rate, before and after suctioning.
5. Suction the "baby's" endotracheal tube.
6. Monitor the "baby's" response and oxygen saturation; adjust inspired oxygen concentration as necessary.
7. Suction the "baby's" mouth.
8. Readjust the "baby's" FiO_2, if it had been increased.

Managing Endotracheal Tubes

In Book I, Resuscitation, you learned how to insert and check for proper placement of an endotracheal tube. You also learned how to secure the tube in place with adhesive tape. If you anticipate that the endotracheal tube will be required for longer than several hours (ie, for a baby requiring mechanical ventilation), the tube should be fixed in place more securely than with tape alone. Be sure the baby is being adequately ventilated and that an assistant is holding the tube in place while it is being secured.

Securing and suctioning an endotracheal tube are 2-person procedures.

Two different methods for long-term stabilization of an endotracheal tube are described. The first uses materials generally available in most hospitals. The second method requires purchase of a commercial stabilizer.

Actions	Remarks

Securing an Endotracheal Tube Without a Commercial Stabilizer

1. Collect the necessary equipment and supplies.

   - Elastoplast elastic bandage
   - 2-0 silk suture on a curved needle
   - Needle holder
   - 1/2-inch adhesive tape
   - Scissors
   - Clear adhesive dressing film

   Only a small rectangular piece (about 1 × 2 inches) will be needed.

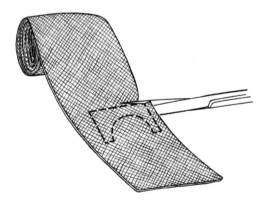

2. Cut a "mustache" from the piece of Elastoplast.

3. Take one stitch through the Elastoplast near the curved edge and make a knot, leaving long lengths of suture on either side of the knot.

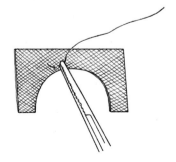

Actions	**Remarks**

Securing an Endotracheal Tube Without a Commercial Stabilizer (continued)

4. Cut off and discard the needle.

5. If the tube was previously taped, remove the tape and ask an assistant to hold the tube in place.

   Note the markings on the tube at the baby's lip. Be sure the tube is held at this position.

6. Cut a piece of clear adhesive dressing in the same size and shape as the Elastoplast. Stick this across the baby's upper lip and on the cheeks near the sides of the mouth.

   Clear adhesive dressings stick well if the
   - Baby's skin is dry
   - Sticky side does not become dusted with glove powder

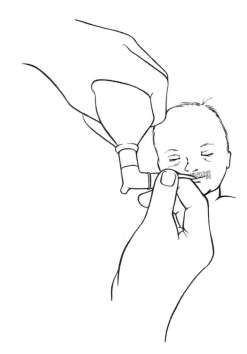

7. Smooth the Elastoplast mustache firmly over the clear adhesive dressing mustache.

8. Be sure the tube is in the proper position.

   - Recheck the markings on the tube at the baby's lip (step 5).

   - Listen with a stethoscope

     - Over both left and right sides of the baby's chest, for equal breath sounds
     - Over the baby's stomach, to be certain the tube has not slipped into the esophagus

Actions	**Remarks**

Securing an Endotracheal Tube Without a Commercial Stabilizer (continued)

9. Tie the tube to the Elastoplast mustache with the suture.

   Tie tightly, but be careful not to constrict the lumen of the tube.

The same type of knot may be used that was used to secure arterial catheters in place (see Book II: Neonatal Care, Umbilical Catheters).

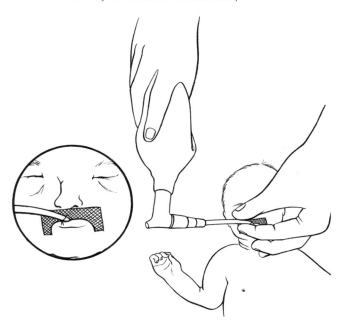

10. Tape the tube in place.

    - Cut 2 pieces of 1/2-inch adhesive tape 4 inches long.
    - Split each piece for half the length.
    - Stick the unsplit section and one tab across the baby's upper lip on top of the Elastoplast. Wrap the other tab around the endotracheal tube.
    - Place the second piece of tape in the reverse direction.

The technique for taping is similar to that described in Book I, Resuscitation, Endotracheal Intubation skill unit.

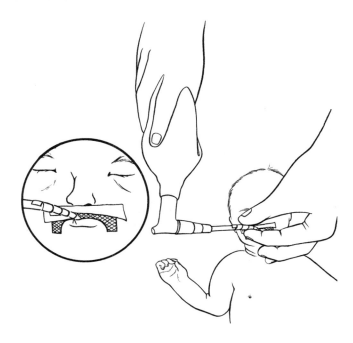

Actions	Remarks

Securing an Endotracheal Tube With a Commercial Stabilizer

1. Be sure the stabilizer fits the brand of endotracheal tube being used.

2. Collect the necessary equipment and supplies.

   - Endotracheal tube holder of the correct size to match the endotracheal tube being used
   - Slip-lock (packaged with holder)
   - Cotton-tipped swab
   - Hemostat

   Holders are manufactured to fit tubes of various sizes (2.5 mm, 3.0 mm, 3.5 mm, 4.0 mm).

3. If the tube was previously taped, remove the tape and ask an assistant to hold the tube in place.

   Note the markings on the tube at the level of the baby's lip. Be sure the tube is held at this position.

4. Peel off the protective backing from the holder and stick the holder to the baby's face with the cylinder located over either side of the mouth.

   The cylinder should be located over one corner of the mouth, while the tube is temporarily held on the other side of the mouth (endotracheal tube not shown in illustration).

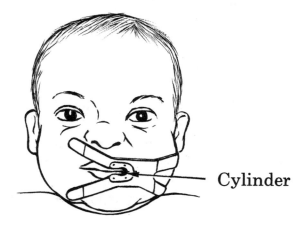

Cylinder

5. Slide the endotracheal tube to the other side of the baby's mouth and slip it into the groove of the cylinder. Be sure to maintain the tube at its original insertion depth (ie, take care not to push the tube in or pull it out slightly as you slide it from one corner of the mouth to the other).

   The height of the cylinder is slightly less than 2 cm, therefore, the top of the cylinder may now be used as a reference point for the markings on the tube (previous marking at the lip plus 2 cm).

Actions	**Remarks**

Securing an Endotracheal Tube With a Commercial Stabilizer (continued)

6. Place the slip-lock around the tube, down over the cylinder, and then turn it to lock in place.

   The slip-lock has a slot that allows it to be placed over the tube from the side.

   Be careful not to position the slip-lock upside down. The side with the smaller diameter should be toward the baby. If positioned correctly, writing imprinted on the top of the slip-lock will be visible.

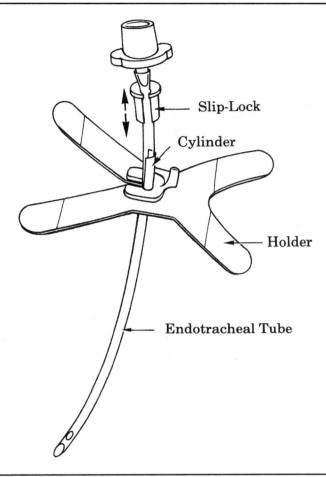

Slip-Lock

Cylinder

Holder

Endotracheal Tube

Checking/Changing Endotracheal Tube Position

1. Obtain a portable chest x-ray to check for tube placement.

   The tube tip should be visible by x-ray just below the level of the clavicles and 1 to 2 cm above the carina (point where the mainstem bronchi branch from the trachea).

2. Adjust the tube position (further out or further in) if necessary.

   Suture and tape method: Remove the adhesive tape, but leave the Elastoplast untouched. You may then be able to slip the tube through the suture. If not, the suture should be cut, a new suture carefully secured to the Elastoplast, retied to the tube, and the tube retaped.

   Commercial stabilizer method: The tube may be adjusted by simply unlocking the slip-lock, sliding the tube the desired distance, then relocking the slip-lock. If the endotracheal tube needs to be replaced, you will usually need to remove and replace the stabilizer too.

Actions	**Remarks**

Checking/Changing Endotracheal Tube Position (continued)

3. Check to be sure the tube has not slipped since the x-ray was obtained.

   - Watch to see if the chest is moving symmetrically.

   - Listen to both sides of the chest for equal breath sounds, and over the stomach, to be sure the tube is not in the esophagus.

   - If in doubt, insert a CO_2 detector or check position with a laryngoscope and obtain another chest x-ray.

Suctioning an Endotracheal Tube

1. Collect the necessary equipment and supplies.

   - Appropriate-sized suction catheter
   - Sterile gloves
   - 1/2-mL sterile saline
   - Suction source and tubing
   - Anesthesia bag with pressure manometer

   Suction catheter sizes for various size endotracheal tubes:

Endotracheal Tube Inner Diameter	*Suction Catheter*
2.5 mm	5F or 6F
3.0 mm	5F or 6F
3.5 mm	6F or 8F
4.0 mm	6F, 8F, or 10F

   If secretions are thin, select a small catheter to decrease the chances of collapsing the lung during suctioning. If secretions are thick, select the largest possible catheter.

2. Plan to suction the endotracheal tube periodically to be sure it is clear for maximum airflow.

   - Initially every 3 to 4 hours for babies with no lung disease.
   - Initially as frequently as every 30 minutes for babies with severe lung disease such as meconium aspiration.
   - Intervals between suctioning may be lengthened as the volume of mucus and debris decline until suctioning may be done only when clinically indicated.

   An endotracheal tube bypasses the baby's normal mechanism to clear the lungs of mucus and debris.

   Listen to the chest with a stethoscope. If coarse ronchi rather than clear breath sounds are heard, the baby may need suctioning.

3. ***Do not suction unnecessarily.***

   If little or no mucus is recovered, blood gases and/or pulse oximetry are stable, and clear breath sounds are heard with a stethoscope, routine suctioning is not required and may be harmful.

Actions	**Remarks**

Suctioning an Endotracheal Tube (continued)

4. Monitor oximetry and adjust inspired oxygen concentration as necessary.

   Suctioning is stressful for a baby and can cause the blood oxygen level to fall temporarily. It is important for you to minimize the degree and duration of that drop.

5. Completely occlude the suction source. Adjust the vacuum to approximately 60 to 80 mm Hg.

6. Connect the hub of an appropriate-sized catheter to the tubing from the suction source.

   Leave the rest of the catheter within the sterile package.

7. Put on a pair of sterile gloves and remove the suction catheter from its package.

   Suctioning should be performed as a sterile procedure.

8. Estimate the length of the endotracheal tube and hold the suction catheter that distance plus 1 cm (1/2 inch) from the tip of the catheter.

   Example: If the ET tube is 12 cm long, hold the suction catheter 13 cm from its tip. Some catheters are made with centimeter marks printed on the catheter. If the endotracheal tube also has centimeter marks, the depth of suctioning can be judged by matching the catheter and endotracheal tube markings.

   The baby should have cardiac and pulse oximetry monitoring during suctioning.

   If the heart rate falls significantly, the baby turns blue, or oxygenation drops dramatically, stop the procedure and assist ventilation with a resuscitation bag and 100% oxygen.

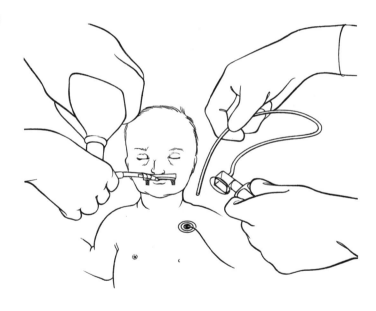

9. Have an assistant disconnect the endotracheal tube from the bag or respirator.

   Suctioning is a 2-person procedure.

10. Quickly insert the suction catheter only to the measured distance (which will push the catheter 1 cm beyond the end of the endotracheal tube). Begin suctioning by occluding the thumbhole on the catheter and continue suctioning as the catheter is withdrawn.

    Stimulation from the catheter tip will probably cause the baby to cough. Avoid excessive stimulation.

11. ***Do not insert the catheter too far.***

    The trachea can be damaged or even perforated by suctioning that is too vigorous.

Actions	**Remarks**

Suctioning an Endotracheal Tube (continued)

12. The assistant should connect the anesthesia bag and deliver several breaths at slightly higher pressures than the baby was receiving prior to suctioning.	Suctioning may cause some collapse of lung segments, which need to be reinflated after the procedure.
13. If significant amounts of material (mucus, meconium, etc) are retrieved, repeat steps 8 through 11, once the baby's oxygenation is stable again.	If the suctioned material is thick, consider instilling 1/2 mL of sterile normal saline down the endotracheal tube. Ask your assistant to give the baby a few bagging breaths, then repeat steps 8 through 11.
14. Gently suction the baby's mouth to clear it of any saliva or mucus.	To avoid contamination of the baby's airway, always suction the mouth *after* the trachea has been suctioned.
15. Return the baby's inflation pressure and inspired oxygen concentration to the pre-suctioning levels.	
16. Reconnect the baby to the ventilator or continue bag-breathing for the baby.	

Unit 7   Surfactant Therapy

Objectives

In this unit you will learn

A. The nature of surfactant deficiency

B. How surfactant deficiency is treated

C. Which babies are likely to benefit from surfactant therapy

D. The recognized complications of giving surfactant

E. The general considerations for administration of commercial preparations of surfactant

Unit 7 Pretest

Before reading the unit, please answer the following questions. Select the *one best* answer to each question (unless otherwise instructed). Record your answers on the answer sheet that is the last page in this book *and* on the test.

1. Natural surfactant

    A. Contains phospholipids and proteins
    B. Raises surface tension in the alveoli
    C. Prevents alveolar collapse during inspiration
    D. Is manufactured in the liver

2. Natural surfactant injected through an endotracheal tube

    A. Spreads very slowly to the lower airways
    B. Is mostly absorbed into the pulmonary circulation and degraded by the liver
    C. Will have a direct effect on alveolar stability
    D. Is most commonly given as a powder

3. Which of the following is an accurate statement about surfactant deficiency?

    A. It is the cause of respiratory distress syndrome.
    B. Incidence increases with increasing gestational age.
    C. It can be treated with intravenous surfactant.
    D. It is only seen in preterm babies.

4. Which of the following babies is at *lowest* risk for developing respiratory distress syndrome?

    A. Baby born at 29 weeks' gestation
    B. Mother has diabetes mellitus
    C. Baby is infected with group B beta hemolytic streptococcus
    D. Mother is infected with HIV

5. Preterm babies who have been stressed in utero have a _____ incidence of respiratory distress syndrome.

    A. Higher
    B. Lower

6. Which of the following is the appropriate method(s) of surfactant administration?

    A. Bolus instillation into the trachea
    B. Intravenous drip
    C. Intratracheal drip
    D. All of the above

7. **True False** All commercial surfactants contain the same components.

8. **True False** Betamethasone or dexamethasone given to a pregnant woman, plus surfactant given to the preterm baby, is more beneficial than surfactant given alone.

9. **True False** By 32 weeks' gestation, approximately 60% of fetuses are producing adequate surfactant to prevent respiratory distress syndrome.

10. **True False** All surfactant components are produced by the lung at the same time during gestation.

11. **True False** Studies have shown that the earlier surfactant is used, the more effective it is.

For each question, please make sure you have marked your answer on the test and on the answer sheet (last page in book). The test is for you; the answer sheet will need to be turned in for continuing education credit.

1. What Is Surfactant?

Surfactant is a complex of substances (phospholipids and proteins) that are essential to normal lung function. The substances are produced by special cells in the lining of the alveoli and are then secreted onto the surface of the alveoli. The surfactant components work together to lower the surface tension at the air-liquid interface, so that the alveoli will remain open and not collapse completely during exhalation.

2. When Is Surfactant Made During Fetal Development?

The various components of the surfactant complex are produced at different stages of fetal development. All components are necessary for normal physiologic function of the complex, but all are not produced and secreted until midway through the third trimester. By 32 weeks' gestation, approximately 60% of fetuses will have adequate surfactant for normal extrauterine respiration.

The surfactant that is secreted into alveoli also appears in the amniotic fluid from fetal respiration, where it can be measured from a sample obtained by amniocentesis. Lecithin and phosphatidyl glycerol (PG) are 2 surfactant phospholipids. Measurement of PG and/or the lecithin/sphingomyelin ratio in amniotic fluid is commonly used to determine fetal lung maturity (Book I, Fetal Age, Growth, and Maturity).

3. What Is Surfactant Deficiency?

Without adequate surfactant, alveoli will collapse during exhalation, causing respiratory distress syndrome (RDS) to develop in the baby (Book II: Neonatal Care, Respiratory Distress). Factors that increase the risk of surfactant deficiency include

A. *Preterm birth:* Surfactant components have not yet been produced by the lung. The more preterm a baby is, the greater the risk of RDS.

B. *Maternal diabetes mellitus:* Excess insulin produced by the fetus in response to high maternal blood glucose inhibits surfactant production (Book I, Fetal Age, Growth, and Maturity).

C. *Pneumonia:* Inflammation of the lung causes leakage of serum proteins into the alveoli; these proteins inhibit surfactant function.

D. *Aspiration syndrome:* Foreign substances, such as meconium, blood, or amniotic fluid aspirated into the alveoli may inactivate surfactant.

Conversely, preterm babies who have had a moderate amount of stress in utero may have a *decreased* incidence of respiratory distress syndrome because the stress may stimulate surfactant production.

4. How Can Surfactant Deficiency Be Treated?

Surfactant deficiency in newborns can be treated by administration of surfactant to the airways of the lung; several liquid surfactant preparations are available commercially. Because of its tendency to spread rapidly, surfactant placed in the trachea will move very quickly throughout the airways of the lungs to have a direct effect on maintaining alveolar stability. In addition, the administered surfactant eventually will be absorbed by the lungs and re-secreted as natural surfactant.

5. Does Maternal Steroid Administration Affect Neonatal Respiratory Distress Syndrome and the Need for Surfactant Therapy?

Administration of steroids (betamethasone or dexamethasone) to the pregnant woman prior to delivery will stimulate fetal surfactant production, thus decreasing the chance of a preterm baby developing RDS. If RDS is present, however, surfactant therapy acts additively with antenatal corticosteroids to reduce the severity of RDS. See Book I, Fetal Age, Growth, Maturity and Book II: Maternal/Fetal, Preterm Labor for more information and recommendations regarding antenatal administration of steroids.

6. Are All Surfactant Preparations the Same?

No. The surfactant preparations that are available commercially are not the same compounds. They can be divided into 2 groups.

A. Natural Surfactants

Survanta, Infasurf, and Curosurf are surfactant preparations that have been extracted from animal lung, although by different methods. These preparations contain all of the surfactant phospholipids and 2 of the 3 proteins, but in different proportions.

B. Synthetic Surfactants

Exosurf and Surfaxin are manufactured from synthetic phospholipids and have added spreading agents or protein analogues. Several of the phospholipids are not present and neither of the preparations contain any of the surfactant-specific proteins.

Each of the commercial preparations has been studied extensively. All have been shown to be effective in treating RDS. While there are relatively minor differences among the natural surfactants, the natural surfactants as a group seem to have a more rapid onset of action and a more striking effect on oxygenation and lung compliance than does synthetic surfactant. No studies have been large enough to demonstrate a clear difference in mortality or chronic lung disease for any of the preparations.

Self-Test

Now answer these questions to test yourself on the information in the last section.

A1. The naturally occurring surfactant complex is composed of 2 groups of substances: _____ and _____.

A2. Surfactant works by _____ surface tension in the alveoli and preventing alveoli from collapsing during _____.

A3. **True** **False** All components of the surfactant complex appear for the first time at 32 weeks' gestation.

A4. **True** **False** A preterm fetus who has been subjected to chronic stress will have a greater chance of developing respiratory distress syndrome.

A5. List 4 factors known to increase the likelihood of a baby developing respiratory problems from surfactant deficiency.

_____

_____

_____

_____

A6. **True** **False** When commercially available surfactant is given through an endotracheal tube, it will eventually be absorbed by the lungs and re-secreted as natural surfactant.

A7. **True** **False** Babies born to women who were given betamethasone or dexamethasone are more likely to require surfactant therapy.

A8. **True** **False** All commercially available surfactants contain the main components of naturally occurring surfactant, but in different proportions.

Check your answers with the list near the end of the unit. Correct any incorrect answers and review the appropriate section in the unit.

7. How Do You Give Surfactant?

All of the surfactant preparations are given directly into a baby's trachea, through an endotracheal tube, although each manufacturer recommends a different administration technique. Survanta, Infasurf, and Curosurf are recommended to be given through a catheter that is inserted into the endotracheal tube. The Exosurf manufacturer recommends giving it through the side port of a special endotracheal tube adapter, and Surfaxin must first be heated in a water bath before administration.

Recommendations regarding the need to divide the dose and to tilt the baby into various positions also differ considerably. No studies have clearly demonstrated any one technique is superior to another. Bolus administration, however, has been shown to be preferable to aerosol or slow-drip administration, although new techniques for aerosol delivery are currently being evaluated.

 Correct endotracheal tube position is very important, to ensure that the surfactant is administered into the trachea and not into one mainstem bronchus and thus into only one lung.

After surfactant administration, the compliance (stiffness) of the lung is likely to change quite rapidly, particularly with the natural surfactants. As compliance improves (lungs become less stiff), you should make corresponding changes in ventilator or bag-breathing pressures. Usually a rapid decrease in peak inspiratory pressure is needed first, but other changes may be needed too.

Monitor oxygen saturation continuously, check arterial blood gases frequently, and adjust the baby's inspired oxygen concentration and inspiratory pressure according to percent saturation and PaO_2 results. Low $PaCO_2$ is also an important indication to decrease peak inspiratory pressure and rate.

 To minimize the chance of a pneumothorax occurring, anticipate likely changes in the baby's lung compliance following surfactant administration.

Make changes in ventilation pressures promptly in response to oxygen saturation and blood gas results.

Following surfactant administration, some experts prefer to continue to bag-breathe for a baby for a brief period, using an anesthesia bag and in-line manometer, rather than reconnecting the baby to a ventilator. Inspiratory pressure is monitored continuously and adjusted immediately according to apparent changes in lung compliance and oxygen saturation readings. Once the oxygen saturation seems to have stabilized, the baby is reconnected to the ventilator with settings that reproduce those used to bag-breathe for the baby. Ventilator settings are likely to need further readjustment, but the rate of change is usually slower than what is needed immediately following the initial dose of surfactant.

8. Which Babies Should Be Treated and When?

Most experts agree that any baby with severe or moderate respiratory distress syndrome should receive surfactant therapy. The earlier surfactant is administered, the more effective it is. Although the optimum timing of administration has not been defined, current recommendations are that surfactant should be given if a baby who has RDS

- Requires endotracheal intubation for respiratory support
- Needs more than 30% to 40% inspired oxygen

There is evidence that babies who are at high risk for developing RDS (eg, those born at 30 weeks' gestation or less) should receive surfactant immediately after birth in an effort to prevent the development of RDS. Several studies have shown that this prophylactic administration of surfactant is more effective than delaying administration until after development of disease. However, because not all preterm babies, even very preterm ones, will develop RDS, prophylaxis will result in unnecessary treatment of some babies.

If surfactant is to be given prophylactically, it is generally agreed that the baby should receive any necessary resuscitation measures prior to surfactant administration, as well as having vital signs stabilized and correct endotracheal tube position ensured. Usually these resuscitative and/or stabilization measures can be accomplished quickly, allowing surfactant to be given within 5 to 10 minutes following birth.

Administration of surfactant after respiratory disease has developed is termed "rescue." Many experts elect to administer surfactant prophylactically to babies born extremely preterm and to use a rescue approach for more mature babies who develop respiratory distress after birth. Some experts advise a modified approach in which surfactant is not given prophylactically, but is given if a preterm baby develops the slightest signs of RDS.

Several reports have suggested that babies, including term babies, with aspiration syndrome, pneumonia, and perhaps "shock lung," may also benefit from surfactant rescue therapy. There is currently insufficient information for this to be a routine recommendation.

9. How Often Should You Give Surfactant?

Depending on the preparation used, if a baby was treated prophylactically or received the first dose soon after birth, a single dose of surfactant will often suffice. However, because surfactant may be absorbed, metabolized, and/or inactivated after administration, repeat doses are sometimes given.

Recommendations regarding repeat doses vary. With *natural surfactants*, if a baby continues to require endotracheal intubation, positive-pressure ventilation, and an inspired oxygen concentration of 30% to 40% or higher, many clinicians will give a repeat dose every 6 to 8 hours, until a maximum of 4 doses has been given. With *synthetic surfactants*, no value of giving more than 2 doses of either Exosurf or Surfaxin has been demonstrated.

10. What Are the Recognized Complications of Surfactant Therapy?

A. Administration to Only One Lung

If surfactant is given into one lung (because the endotracheal tube was too low), the baby may develop a marked compliance difference between the 2 lungs. This can result in major problems with ventilation, with the treated lung becoming over-inflated while the other lung cannot be inflated well at the same inflation pressure. Before administering surfactant, confirm correct endotracheal tube position by

- Visualizing the vocal cord stripe on the endotracheal tube before removing the laryngoscope
- Listening with a stethoscope over both sides of the chest for equal breath sounds
- Obtaining a chest x-ray to confirm tube placement (usually not done when surfactant is given in the delivery room)

B. Development of Air Leaks

If bagging or ventilator pressures are not decreased as lung compliance changes, the baby may develop a pneumothorax or pulmonary interstitial emphysema (bubbles of air within the lung tissue).

C. Endotracheal Tube Becomes Slippery

The phospholipids in surfactant make it very slippery. After surfactant administration, the endotracheal tube, the tube connector, and the baby's airway may also be slippery, perhaps making tube adjustment or reintubation difficult. Be certain all connections are tight and all adjustments have been made *before* administering surfactant.

D. Endotracheal Tube Becomes Blocked With the Surfactant Solution

Sometimes, during surfactant administration, the surfactant solution will back up into the endotracheal tube and prevent gas movement. If liquid is seen to be blocking the tube, use slightly higher pressure and longer inflation time for several breaths until the tube clears. If the baby's condition deteriorates despite these measures, the surfactant can be suctioned from the tube or the tube can be replaced.

E. Severe Oxygen Desaturation Occurs During Administration

Babies with severe RDS may not tolerate the introduction of liquid into their endotracheal tubes. Most manufacturers recommend that the dose be divided into 2 or 4 portions. After each partial dose, the baby should be ventilated for a few minutes, until the oxygen saturation is greater than 90%, before the next partial dose is given.

11. Should Surfactant Always Be Given in an Intensive Care Facility?

Surfactant administration requires considerable expertise with endotracheal intubation and mechanical ventilation. Babies who require surfactant usually will also require intensive care for management of other immature organ systems, in addition to the lungs. It is recommended* that surfactant therapy be given only in hospitals appropriately equipped and staffed for the management of low birth weight infants, including use of mechanical ventilators.

An appropriate exception may be administering surfactant, in a non-intensive care setting, to a baby with severe RDS for whom there may be a significant delay in transport to an intensive care nursery. If surfactant is to be given under these conditions, it should be administered by individuals skilled in endotracheal intubation who have reviewed in detail the specific recommended techniques for administering the commercial surfactant being used. In addition, familiarity and skill with rapid lowering of inspiratory pressures with either bag-breathing or ventilator adjustment, following surfactant administration, is important.

---

*American Academy of Pediatrics, American College of Obstetricians and Gynecologists. *Guidelines for Perinatal Care,* 5th ed. Elk Grove Village, IL: American Academy of Pediatrics; 2002:250–251.

Self-Test

Now answer these questions to test yourself on the information in the last section.

B1. Which of the following techniques have been shown to be important for administering *all* commercially available surfactant products?

Yes   No

____ ____   Administration through a special endotracheal tube connector, which has a side port
____ ____   Careful positioning of the endotracheal tube tip in the midtrachea
____ ____   Turning the baby 360°
____ ____   Monitoring oxygen saturation during administration
____ ____   Anticipating changes in lung compliance and adjusting ventilation pressures accordingly

B2. **True   False**   Studies have shown that surfactant given immediately after birth is more effective than waiting until a baby develops significant respiratory disease.

B3. With natural surfactants, many clinicians recommend that a baby who continues to have significant respiratory distress after initial surfactant administration be re-treated in _____ hours.

B4. List 4 possible complications of surfactant therapy.

_____

_____

_____

_____

Check your answers with the list near the end of the unit. Correct any incorrect answers and review the appropriate section in the unit.

These are the answers to the self-test questions. Please check them with the answers you gave and review the information in the unit wherever necessary.

A1.   Phospholipids and proteins
A2.   Lowering
         Exhalation
A3.   False   The various components of surfactant are first produced at different times during gestation. By 32 weeks, 60% of fetuses have adequate surfactant for normal extrauterine respiration.
A4.   False   Fetuses subjected to chronic stress are *less* likely to develop respiratory distress syndrome.
A5.   Preterm birth
         Maternal diabetes mellitus
         Pneumonia
         Aspiration syndrome
A6.   True
A7.   False   Antenatal steroids and neonatal surfactant have an additive effect on preventing respiratory distress syndrome.
A8.   False   Survanta, Infasurf, and Curosurf contain all of the natural phospholipids but only 2 of the 3 proteins; Exosurf and Surfaxin contain several synthetic phospholipids and no surfactant-specific protein.

B1.   Which of the following techniques have been shown to be important for administering *all* commercially available surfactant products?

         Yes   No
         ___   _x_   Administration through a special endotracheal tube connector, which has a side port
         _x_   ___   Careful positioning of the endotracheal tube tip in the midtrachea
         ___   _x_   Turning the baby 360°
         _x_   ___   Monitoring oxygen saturation during administration
         _x_   ___   Anticipating changes in lung compliance and adjusting ventilation pressures accordingly

B2.   True
B3.   6 to 8 hours
B4.   Any 4 of the following:
   • Administration to one lung
   • Development of air leaks (pneumothorax, etc)
   • Endotracheal tube becomes slippery
   • Endotracheal tube becomes blocked with surfactant
   • Severe oxygen desaturation occurs during administration

Unit 7 Posttest

Without referring back to the information in the unit, please answer the following questions. Select the **one best** answer to each question (unless otherwise instructed). Record your answers on the answer sheet that is the last page in this book *and* on the test.

1. Natural surfactant

    A. Prevents air trapping during expiration
    B. Raises surface tension in the alveolus
    C. Is manufactured in the white blood cells
    D. Contains lecithin and phosphatidyl glycerol

2. Which of the following babies is at *lowest* risk for developing respiratory distress syndrome?

    A. Baby born at 30 weeks' gestation
    B. Mother has diabetes mellitus
    C. Baby aspirated meconium
    D. Mother is a substance user

3. Surfactant in the delivery room

    A. Should be given after vital signs have stabilized
    B. Requires a higher dose than if given later
    C. Should always be given before the first breath
    D. Should not be given; it is always better to wait until the baby develops respiratory distress syndrome

4. All of the following are recognized as possible complications of surfactant therapy *except*

    A. Blockage of endotracheal tube with surfactant solution
    B. Pneumothorax from rapidly improving compliance
    C. Oxygen desaturation during surfactant administration
    D. Anaphylactic reaction to the surfactant protein

5. Repeat doses of surfactant

    A. Are always needed, because administered surfactant is absorbed and metabolized
    B. Are indicated if a baby remains intubated and continues to require more than 30% to 40% inspired oxygen
    C. Should be given every hour for 4 doses
    D. Are contraindicated

6. Decreased surfactant function has been associated with all of the following neonatal conditions *except*

    A. Meconium aspiration syndrome
    B. Bacterial pneumonia
    C. Respiratory distress syndrome
    D. Transient tachypnea of the newborn

7. **True   False**   Babies who have been stressed in utero should routinely receive a prophylactic dose of surfactant.

8. **True   False**   The various components of surfactant are made at various times during gestation.

9. **True   False**   Studies have shown that slow infusion of surfactant into the trachea may be more effective than giving a rapid bolus.

10. **True   False**   By 32 weeks' gestation, more than 90% of fetuses have produced adequate surfactant to prevent respiratory distress syndrome.

For each question, please make sure you have marked your answer on the test and on the answer sheet (last page in book). The test is for you; the answer sheet will need to be turned in for continuing education credit.

Skill Unit   Surfactant Administration

There are several different commercial surfactant preparations. Each has been shown to be effective in preventing and treating neonatal respiratory distress syndrome, although the techniques for administration vary significantly among the different preparations. Each manufacturer has prepared detailed instructions regarding the recommended method for administering that company's particular product. These instructions are available in written and video formats. You may be asked to participate in a skill session to practice surfactant administration according to the methods recommended for the surfactant chosen for use in your hospital.

Because administration techniques vary considerably for the different products, it is recommended that your hospital use only one brand of surfactant, and all staff become skilled in using that particular product. Switching between brands makes it more difficult to become skilled in the use of each product and increases the risk of errors in administration.

Objectives

In this unit you will learn to

A. Provide long-term care for an at-risk infant who remains in your hospital for longer than several days.

B. Provide continuity of care for an at-risk infant who returns from an intensive care nursery to your hospital.

C. Plan for the discharge of an at-risk infant.

Unit 8 Pretest

Before reading the unit, please answer the following questions. Select the *one best* answer to each question (unless otherwise instructed). Record your answers on the answer sheet that is the last page in this book *and* on the test.

1. A term baby with short bowel syndrome recently returned to your nursery from a regional intensive care nursery. Which of the following is *least* important for you to monitor in this baby?

    A. Urine pH
    B. Weight gain
    C. Frequency of stools
    D. Blood electrolytes

2. Two weeks ago a 1,500-g (3 lb, 5 oz) preterm baby returned to your hospital after 3 weeks in a regional intensive care nursery. The parents live in your town and have visited the baby once in the past 2 weeks. What would you do?

    Yes **No**
    ___ ___ Request consultation from social service department staff.
    ___ ___ Call the parents and chat with them about their baby.
    ___ ___ Begin making plans for the baby to be sent to a foster home.

3. Which of the following babies is at *highest* risk for developing hydrocephalus?

    A. Term baby treated for hypoglycemia
    B. 1,000-g (2 lb, 4 oz) preterm infant requiring assisted ventilation
    C. 36-week gestational age baby who received an exchange transfusion
    D. 1,800-g (4 lb) baby born at 40 weeks' gestation

4. All of the following regarding retinopathy of prematurity are correct *except*

    A. Laser photocoagulation may be helpful in reducing poor visual outcome from retinopathy of prematurity.
    B. Retinopathy of prematurity is unlikely to develop in babies born at term.
    C. Mild-to-moderate retinopathy of prematurity may completely resolve.
    D. All preterm babies with a PaO_2 greater than 100 mm Hg will develop retinopathy of prematurity.

5. A preterm baby requires assisted ventilation and several weeks of intensive care at a regional center. Now the baby is stable, weighs 1,500 g (3 lb, 5 oz), has no respiratory distress, and is returning to your nursery for further weight gain. Which of the following should be done for this baby?

    Yes **No**
    ___ ___ Measure baby's head circumference once a week.
    ___ ___ Start the baby on phenobarbital.
    ___ ___ Weigh the baby daily.
    ___ ___ Give Imferon intramuscularly.
    ___ ___ Check the baby's hematocrit at least once a week.
    ___ ___ Attach the baby to a cardiac or respiratory monitor.

6. **True   False**   A 4,540-g (10 lb) baby has seizures controlled on a certain drug dose. By the time the baby reaches 9,070 g (20 lb), he should be receiving twice as much medication.

7. **True   False**   When a baby reaches 1,500 g (3 lb, 5 oz) and respiratory disease has resolved, it is safe to assume the baby will not have an apneic spell.

8. **True   False**   Nipple feedings should be used for any baby who has a gag reflex and can suck on a nipple.

9. **True   False**   Babies with chronic lung disease can grow completely new, healthy lung tissue.

10. **True   False**   After a baby with hydrocephalus has a shunt placed, it is no longer necessary to measure the baby's head circumference.

11. **True   False**   It is a good sign if a baby with congenital heart disease gains 60 g (2 oz) or more per day for several days in a row.

12. **True   False**   Babies requiring theophylline or caffeine to control apneic spells may have the drug stopped and be sent home the next day, as long as they have reached a weight of 1,800 g (4 lb).

13. **True   False**   Any baby with short bowel syndrome will need an ostomy (colostomy or ileostomy) for the rest of his or her life.

14. All of the following are common causes of anemia in preterm infants *except*
    A. Blood taken from the baby for laboratory tests
    B. Drop in hemoglobin or hematocrit that occurs after birth
    C. Bronchopulmonary dysplasia

15. Which of the following should you do when supplementing a baby's nipple feedings with tube feedings given through a nasogastric or orogastric tube?
    A. Feed the baby as much as he or she will take by nipple, then insert a feeding tube and give the remainder of the feeding through the tube.
    B. Feed the baby as much as he or she will take by nipple while a feeding tube is in place, then give the remainder of the feeding through the tube.

16. All of the following steps are important in weaning a baby from an incubator *except*
    A. Putting a stocking cap on the baby's head
    B. Wrapping the baby in blankets
    C. Recording the baby's daily weight during the weaning period
    D. Adjusting the room temperature to neutral thermal environment during the weaning period

17. Indicate which of the following things should be routinely checked for a hospitalized baby with congenital heart disease and congestive heart failure:

Yes	No	
___	___	Blood electrolytes
___	___	Volume of urine output
___	___	Stool pH
___	___	Hematocrit
___	___	Weight gain
___	___	Blood calcium

For each question, please make sure you have marked your answer on the test and on the answer sheet (last page in book). The test is for you; the answer sheet will need to be turned in for continuing education credit.

1. Which Babies Require Continuing Care?

A. Babies Who Need Additional Weight Gain

Preterm babies who have recovered from their initial illness are now at risk but stable, and need continued hospitalization until they gain adequate weight to be discharged.

B. Babies Who Need Special Monitoring

Any baby who has recovered from an initial illness but has a special medical problem that requires continued hospitalization for special monitoring or intervention.

Note: Babies with family problems should be identified *as early as possible* so social issues do not become a cause for delayed discharge and prolonged hospitalization and a home situation can be identified that best meets the baby's needs.

2. What Is Continuing Care?

At-risk infants, even though they are not sick, require certain daily caretaking activities and certain types of monitoring. The following is a list of routine care practices needed for infants requiring continuing care.

A. Temperature Control

Any preterm baby requires an incubator adjusted to the appropriate neutral thermal environment (NTE), until the baby weighs approximately 1,600 to 1,700 g (3 lb, 8 1/2 oz–3 lb, l2 oz). At that weight most stable babies can be weaned to a crib.

B. Feeding

Any baby less than 32 to 34 weeks' gestational age requires tube feedings. After this gestational age, if the baby has a gag reflex and is not sick, nipple feedings may be started. If a baby tires quickly with nipple feedings, tube feedings may be used to supplement.

C. Assessment of Growth
- *Weight:* It is important for a baby to have consistent weight gain to be discharged. Daily weights should be obtained and recorded on a growth chart that shows the normal weight gain for preterm babies.
- *Head circumference:* Head circumference should be measured and recorded every week.
  - Occasionally, babies (particularly if they had been critically ill and/or of very low birth weight) will develop a rapidly and abnormally enlarging head.
  - Sometimes babies who experienced severe perinatal compromise will show very poor head growth.
- *Length:* Length should be measured and recorded every week. The most accurate measurement requires that 2 individuals assist in measuring a baby.

D. Monitoring for Apnea
- *Cardiorespiratory monitors:* Although different centers use various criteria, many believe that monitoring for apnea is important until a baby

  1. Weighs 1,800 g (4 lb)
  2. Has reached a gestational age of 35 weeks or more
  3. Has had no apnea for 7 to 8 consecutive days

  A heart rate monitor will detect bradycardia that develops as a result of apnea. A respiratory monitor will detect the apneic spell itself. (See Book I, Unit 4 skill.)

- *Medications:* Some babies may have been given drugs, such as theophylline or caffeine, to reduce the number of apneic attacks. Any baby on such medication should have blood samples obtained to check the blood levels of the medication.

E. Monitoring for Anemia

Almost all preterm babies will develop anemia at some time prior to their discharge from the hospital. Blood samples should be obtained periodically to monitor hematocrit.

F. Administering Immunizations
- Very preterm or chronically ill infants who require prolonged hospitalization should be immunized. Most infants, including preterm infants, who are 8 weeks postnatal age respond appropriately to immunizations.

  Administration of the following vaccines should be considered for *all babies* at 8 weeks postnatal age, *regardless of their degree of prematurity*:
  - Diphtheria, tetanus, acellular pertussis (DTaP)
  - Haemophilus influenzae Type b conjugate
  - Enhanced inactivated poliovirus (IPV)
  - Pneumococcal conjugate vaccine (PCV)

- Administration of palivizumab (Synagis) is appropriate for many, but not all, preterm babies and babies with chronic lung disease.

- Administration of hepatitis B vaccine should follow the schedule outlined in Book II: Neonatal Care, Infections.

G. Screening for Hearing Deficits

Preterm and sick infants are at risk for hearing deficits. These infants should have a hearing screen before discharge.

Universal screening of all neonates, whether sick, at risk, or well, is recommended and is mandated in most states.

H. Screening for Retinopathy of Prematurity (ROP)

Preterm babies are at risk for ROP. Details and criteria for ROP screening are described in section 4H.

I. Late Head Ultrasound

Most preterm babies born at less than 30 weeks' gestation will have had a cranial ultrasound examination during their acute illness. Current recommendations include a repeat head ultrasound at 36 to 40 weeks' postmenstrual age to detect late development of unsuspected intraventricular hemorrhage, increase in size of the ventricles, and/or periventricular leukomalacia, a risk factor for cerebral palsy.

J. Sleep Position

There is strong evidence that prone (on the stomach) sleeping increases the risk of sudden infant death syndrome (SIDS). While there are often good reasons for prone positioning during acute care, continuing care babies should be placed on their backs for sleep. This will get them accustomed to the sleeping position that will be safest at home, and will encourage parents to put their baby "back to sleep" after discharge. With rare exceptions, babies should be placed supine (on the back) for sleep after discharge home.

K. Assessment of Family

The birth of a preterm and/or sick infant often causes emotional and economic stresses, even within a very stable family. Young parents, single mothers, and parents with little or no caregiving experience and skills have additional stresses.

Extensive teaching and careful observation of maternal-infant and paternal-infant interaction are essential. Family visiting patterns and interactions should be observed and recorded. Early identification of problems is important so interventions can be designed and implemented. A comprehensive, proactive approach to family care is important.

3. What Is Developmental Care?

Much interest has centered on modifying the nursery environment, to reduce light, noise, handling, and interrupted sleep when providing care to sick and at-risk infants. These measures have come to be lumped under the term "developmental care," and have been used for acutely ill infants and for babies needing continuing care.

Many developmental care measures make intuitive sense, and some are particularly welcomed by parents. Large, well-designed studies are needed to identify what, if anything, actually makes a difference in neonatal outcome before specific recommendations can be made regarding these care measures.

The staff in some newborn intensive care units believe in nursing babies in a relatively constant low-light environment while they are extremely immature and critically ill. As these babies approach term and are getting ready for discharge, they should be exposed to the day-night light variation they will encounter at home.

Self-Test

Now answer these questions to test yourself on the information in the last section.

A1. Give 2 reasons a baby may need continuing care.

1. _____

2. _____

A2. List at least 7 basic components of continuing care for preterm infants.

1. _____

2. _____

3. _____

4. _____

5. _____

6. _____

7. _____

A3. What are 3 important ways to assess the growth of babies requiring continuing care?

1. _____

2. _____

3. _____

A4. Preterm babies who need continuing care should be monitored for _____ until they weigh more than

_____ g, have reached a gestational age of _____ weeks, and have had no apneic spells for

_____ consecutive days.

A5. **True   False**   Most infants respond to immunizations when they reach 8 weeks postnatal age, regardless of their gestational age at birth.

Check your answers with the list that follows the Recommended Routines. Correct any incorrect answers and review the appropriate section in the unit.

4. How Do You Provide Care for the Stable Preterm Infant?

A. Temperature Control

Babies less than 1,600 to 1,700 g (3 lb, 8 1/2 oz–3 lb, 12 oz) should be kept in an incubator in the appropriate NTE. When they reach a weight of approximately 1,600 to 1,700 g you may begin to wean them from the incubator to a crib.

Follow these steps to wean a baby from an incubator to a crib.

Step 1.　Wrap the baby with blankets. Put a stocking cap on the baby's head. Reduce the heat in the incubator. Monitor the baby's temperature.

Step 2.　If the baby's temperature is stable after 8 hours, open the portholes of the incubator. Monitor the baby's temperature.

Step 3.　If the baby's temperature is stable after 24 hours, place the baby in a crib. Monitor the baby's temperature.

Note:　If the baby becomes cold (temperature <36.5°C or 97.7°F) at any time, add more cover, check for abnormal routes of heat loss, or go back one step.

What is kangaroo care?

Kangaroo care means skin-to-skin contact between a baby's body and a parent's chest. This may provide sufficient thermal support for a baby to maintain a normal body temperature while outside an incubator. The baby should be naked, except for a diaper, and in direct contact with the bare skin of the parent's chest. The baby should wear a cap and be covered with a blanket, placed over both the baby and the parent's chest.

Note:　Any benefits of kangaroo care have been shown to diminish dramatically if the baby is on the parent's chest for only a few minutes. If a parent has only a short time to spend with the baby, at a particular visit, moving the baby for this brief period is not recommended, especially if the baby is small and is attached to a number of monitors, intravenous lines, and other equipment.

If a breastfeeding mother does not wish to provide kangaroo care, put a cap on the baby and wrap the baby in extra blankets. It may also be possible to use a radiant warmer positioned over the baby and mother.

In all situations when a baby is outside an incubator, the baby's temperature should be monitored frequently.

What can go wrong?

The baby may have a normal temperature but be using a lot of calories to keep warm. This may cause the baby to lose weight or fail to gain weight. Any baby who has just been weaned to a crib who loses weight for 2 to 3 days in a row should be placed back in an incubator.

Caution: Weight loss may occur for other reasons too. You should consider

- Checking for infection
- Assessing feeding pattern and caloric intake
- Checking blood pH to detect acidosis

B. Feeding

Gestational Age: Babies less than 32 to 34 weeks' gestation should be fed with tube feedings. To determine a baby's current gestational age, take the gestational age at birth and add the number of weeks that have passed since birth.

Begin to feed by nipple when a baby

1. Reaches a gestational age of 32 to 34 weeks

2. Has a gag reflex

3. Is not sick

Feeding may be from a bottle, or by breast if the mother desires to breastfeed. Babies who will be breastfeeding may be permitted to explore the breast during kangaroo care, even if they are less than 32 weeks' gestational age. They generally will not latch on to the breast, and even if they aspirate a small amount of breast milk, it will generally not be toxic to the lungs.

Sucking on a pacifier may be used during tube feeding. This has been shown to aid in gastric motility.

Temperature Control: Some infants may be ready to feed by mouth before they are able to control their temperatures outside an incubator. If an infant weighs less than 1,600 to 1,700 g, but otherwise meets criteria for oral feedings, the feedings may be given in the incubator.

Infant Fatigue: Frequently, babies tire when they first start to feed by nipple. For this reason it is often necessary to *alternate* feedings by mouth with tube feedings or to *supplement* feedings taken by mouth with tube feedings.

Note: You may leave the feeding tube in place during a nipple feeding, but never insert it immediately after a feeding. This may cause the baby to vomit and aspirate milk into the lungs.

 Wait at least 1 hour after a feeding before inserting a feeding tube.

- To **alternate** feedings by mouth with tube feedings, follow these steps.

  Step 1. Give the baby the full feeding by tube (nasogastric or orogastric tube).

  Step 2. At the time of the next feeding (2–3 hours later), give the baby the feeding by nipple (breast or bottle).

Step 3.   Give the next feeding by tube.

Step 4.   Repeat the previous cycles for 24 hours. If the baby is taking feedings well by mouth, increase the number of nipple feedings and decrease an equal number of tube feedings until the baby is taking all feedings by mouth.

Some babies will be unable to take the entire amount of a feeding by mouth and will require supplemental feedings.

• To **supplement** partial oral feedings with tube feedings, follow these steps.

Step 1.   Give the baby the full feeding by tube. Leave the tube in place.

Step 2.   At the time of the next feeding (2–3 hours later), give the baby as much of the scheduled feeding by mouth as the baby will tolerate.

Step 3.   Subtract the amount the baby took by mouth from the total amount of the planned feeding. The amount that remains is the amount that should now be given through the tube.

Example
• The planned feeding is 40 mL every 3 hours.
• The baby takes 20 mL by mouth.
• 40 mL–20 mL = 20 mL of the feeding that has not been taken.
• Give the remaining 20 mL to the baby through the feeding tube.

As a baby becomes less tired during feedings, the amount taken by nipple will increase. Do not force a baby to take more by mouth than the baby is capable of eating easily. This just tires the baby and makes it less likely that the next feeding by nipple will go well.

Note: Other feeding methods, such as cup feeding and finger feeding, have been used. These practices should be considered experimental until more information is available regarding their safety and effectiveness.

C.   Assessment of Growth

Weight: Although many preterm babies will need to remain in the nursery until a weight of approximately 2,000 g (4 lb, 7 oz) is reached, some infants who meet all other discharge criteria may be discharged at weights of 1,800 g or below. Stable preterm babies should demonstrate steady weight gain of approximately 20 to 30 g (2/3–l oz) every day.

Many preterm babies are changed from a 24 kcal/oz to a 22 kcal/oz formula when they reach approximately 1,800 g. Babies receiving breast milk may also have supplements added to breast milk to increase the caloric density and vitamin content. See Book II: Neonatal Care, Feeding for additional information about feeding preterm infants, and their vitamin and iron requirements.

It is important to weigh a baby daily. Daily weights should be recorded on a chart that shows the growth of normal preterm infants (Book II: Neonatal Care, Feeding). This will allow you to detect whether the baby is growing like other preterm babies of the same birth weight and age, or if the baby is growing faster or more slowly than expected.

If the baby loses weight several days in a row, you should think

- Is the baby getting adequate calories?

- Is the baby cold?

- Does the baby have a low pH?

- Is the baby infected?

Example

- Baby Crosby is a preterm baby who was transferred back to your hospital when he was 14 days old. His growth chart was sent with him.

- Several days after arrival at your hospital, daily weights show Baby Crosby to be gaining less than 20 to 30 g/day. His growth is no longer following the curve on the chart.

- You examine the baby and find that his vital signs, color, activity, and feeding pattern are all normal. You check the amount of calories he is receiving and find it is adequate.

- Baby Crosby is being weaned from his incubator. You note that for the past several shifts he has been slightly cold with an axillary temperature of 36.4°C (98.0°F).

- You place him back in the incubator for several days. His weight gain gradually returns to normal and again follows the line that other babies of his birth weight follow.

Head Circumference: It is important to measure the head circumferences of babies requiring continuing care. Head size for some babies will increase more rapidly than normal, while for other babies head growth will be less than normal.

- *Increased Head Growth/Hydrocephalus*

  Babies of very low weight or those who were critically ill are at highest risk for developing hydrocephalus. Those with a history of intraventricular bleeding are the babies most likely to develop hydrocephalus.

  Because the normal increase in head size is only a very small amount each day, head circumference is usually measured on a weekly (not daily) basis. Normally, a preterm baby's head circumference will increase between 0.5 and 1.0 cm each week.

  Babies with hydrocephalus may have

  - Rapidly increasing head circumference (>1.25 cm/week)

  - Bulging fontanels

- Eyes that look downward ("sunsetting eyes")
- Prominent veins over the scalp
- Increased irritability
- Persistent vomiting

 If you note any of these signs, the baby should be observed very carefully and evaluated by ultrasonography for possible hydrocephalus.

- *Decreased Head Growth*

    Head size for some babies will *not* increase as expected. These babies may have had severe perinatal compromise or a congenital infection. Rarely, they may have premature closure of the cranial sutures and fusion of the cranial bones. They should be evaluated by ultrasonography. Imaging studies, such as computed tomography scan and magnetic resonance imaging, may be indicated. Consult your regional center.

    If head growth is very poor, the family should be counseled regarding the possibility of developmental compromise and the infant's developmental progress followed with regular, detailed evaluations.

    Length: It is important to measure a baby's length on a weekly basis. Normally a baby's length will increase approximately 0.5 cm/week.

    If length is not increasing, the baby likely has inadequate caloric intake. Less common causes for poor increase in length include malabsorption or rickets.

D. Monitoring for Apnea

1. Which Babies Should Be Monitored?

    Preterm babies, and sick babies of any gestational age, may have apneic spells. For this reason, they require electronic monitoring of heart or respiratory rate. Babies in the following groups should be monitored:

    - All preterm babies less than 1,800 g (4 lb)
    - All babies less than 35 weeks' gestational age
    - Any baby who has had an apneic spell
    - All sick babies

2. How Long Should These Babies Be Monitored?

    - *Preterm babies* should be electronically monitored until they are apnea-free and have reached a
        - Weight of 1,800 g
        and
        - Gestational age of 35 weeks or more

195

- *Babies who have had an apneic spell,* regardless of weight or gestational age, should be electronically monitored until apnea-free.

The specific length of monitoring time is controversial. Most experts agree that monitoring until a baby is apnea-free for 7 to 8 consecutive days is adequate. (See the following information if medication is required to treat frequent apnea episodes.)

3. How Do You Monitor a Baby Receiving Medications to Prevent Apnea?

Some babies have such frequent episodes of apnea that medications (theophylline, caffeine) are used to decrease the number of apneic spells by stimulating the central nervous system.

 No baby should be given these drugs (caffeine, theophylline) until evaluated for the cause of apnea.

Only babies with "apnea of prematurity" should receive these medications, and then only if the episodes are frequent and severe and do not respond to other treatments.

If a baby referred to you is receiving theophylline or caffeine, you should

- Provide continuous electronic cardiorespiratory monitoring. (See Book I, Unit 4 skill.)

- Obtain blood samples regularly to determine the blood level of the drug.

You need to check drug levels because the correct dose is highly variable in small babies. Too much medication in the blood can lead to an increase in heart rate and vomiting; too little medication can lead to an increase in apneic spells.

4. How Long Does a Baby Require Medication to Treat Apnea?

Most preterm babies stop having frequent apneic spells when they reach a weight of approximately 1,800 g (4 lb). Regardless of a baby's weight, the medication should be stopped when apneic spells have decreased to only 1 to 2 mild spells a day. This will allow time for all of the drug to be metabolized and removed from the baby's body to determine if the baby has apneic spells when the drug is no longer present in the blood.

Before discharge, the baby should have a blood level that shows only minimal traces of the drug, *followed by* 7 to 8 consecutive days without an apneic spell.

Most experts are reluctant to discharge babies receiving theophylline or caffeine except in very rare, special cases and with very careful follow-up arrangements among you, the family, and the regional center. Babies who are discharged on theophylline or caffeine and not followed carefully may eventually outgrow their original drug dose, resulting in a low blood level of the medication. They may then have a serious apneic spell at home.

5. When Can a Baby Who Has Had Apnea Go Home?

- *Predischarge preparation*
  Apnea may lead to hypoxia and bradycardia. If a spell is severe and goes undetected, some babies will die.

  In general, however, if a baby is off medication and has had no apnea for 7 to 8 consecutive days, it is very unlikely there will be a severe apneic spell at home.

  Therefore, babies who have had apnea may be discharged home when the baby

  - Weighs 1,800 g (4 lb) or more
  - Has reached a gestational age of 35 weeks or more
  - Has had no apneic attacks for 7 to 8 consecutive days (If a medication was used to treat apnea, then the baby's blood should be tested and shown to be drug-free, followed by 7 to 8 consecutive apnea-free days)
  - Any other problems have been resolved

  OR

- *Home apnea monitoring*
  Occasionally some babies are sent home on apnea monitors. These may include babies who have

  - Demonstrated apnea despite weighing more than 1,800 g and reaching a gestational age of 35 weeks or more

  or

  - Technology-dependent infants who have abnormal regulation of breathing or with symptomatic chronic lung disease

  Discharging a baby with home apnea monitoring requires careful coordination among the family, the regional center staff, and you. The family must have had good instruction in use of the monitor and CPR training. The monitor company must be available to assist the family and care for the monitor. The practice of home monitoring is very controversial.

 Discharge of a baby to home monitoring requires extremely careful follow-up. Consult your regional center staff about these special situations.

E. Monitoring for Anemia

1. How Do You Monitor a Baby's Anemia?

   The baby's hematocrit or hemoglobin should be checked every 1 to 2 weeks. If the hematocrit is less than 25%, it should be checked every 3 to 4 days.

2. What Degree of Anemia Is Dangerous?

   Most babies do not have problems until the hematocrit is less than 25%. If the hematocrit is less than 25%, you should look for these signs

- Sustained increase in heart rate (>160 beats/minute)
- Sustained increase in respiratory rate (>60 breaths/minute)
- Onset of apneic spells or an increase in apneic spells
- Failure to feed well and gain weight

3. What Do You Do If a Baby Who Is Anemic Develops Signs of Anemia?

The baby may need a blood transfusion, or an addition or change in medication. Discuss the best treatment for each specific baby with your regional center staff.

Because of concern for transmission of infections (human immunodeficiency virus, cytomegalovirus, hepatitis) by blood transfusions, many experts recommend transfusing anemic infants only if they are clearly symptomatic from anemia. Before giving a transfusion, you should inform the baby's parents, discuss the risks and benefits of transfusion with them, and obtain a signed consent from them.

Note: Some regional centers give erythropoietin to stimulate red blood cell formation. If you receive a baby who is on this medication, consult with the regional center staff about dosage, duration of therapy, monitoring, and iron supplementation.

4. Why Does a Baby Require Iron?

Preterm babies are born with insufficient iron stores for their subsequent growth. Preterm and sick babies are also at risk for developing anemia due to

- Blood taken from the baby for various laboratory tests
- Normal drop in hemoglobin or hematocrit that occurs in all infants during the first several weeks after birth
- Iron deficiency
- A combination of these factors

A baby transferred back to your hospital may have some degree of anemia and will likely be receiving supplemental iron.

5. How Is Supplemental Iron Provided?

Additional iron may be provided through the use of commercially available, iron-fortified formulas for formula-fed infants or with iron supplements for breastfed infants.

A normal dose is 2 mg of elemental iron per kilogram per day. This amount is provided in iron-fortified formulas when a formula-fed baby is taking full feedings. If a baby is very iron deficient, 5 to 6 mg of elemental iron per kilogram per day may be required.

If supplements are used, whether for breastfed babies or for a baby with severe iron deficiency, liquid ferrous sulfate given daily is started at 6 to 8 weeks of age and when the baby is tolerating feedings (Book II: Neonatal Care, Feeding).

Note: Infants transfused multiple times (>5 transfusions) are usually not iron deficient. However, if follow-up monitoring for anemia is likely to be erratic, these infants should also be discharged on iron supplementation.

F. Administering Immunizations

Hepatitis B vaccine should be given according to the schedule in Book II: Neonatal Care, Infections. For babies returning to your hospital after a period of intensive care, you will need to determine which doses have already been given and continue the schedule recommended for the baby's age, weight, and maternal hepatitis B surface antigen status.

Palivizumab (Synagis): The American Academy of Pediatrics (AAP) recommends that palivizumab be given before discharge and then monthly during respiratory syncytial virus (RSV) season to babies in the groups listed below. RSV season usually runs October through April, but may start earlier or end later in certain areas.

- Infants younger than 24 months of age who have received therapy for chronic lung disease within 6 months before the start of the RSV season.

- Infants younger than 12 months of age if they were born at less than 29 weeks' gestation.

- Infants younger than 6 months of age if they were born at 29 to 32 weeks' gestation.

- Infants younger than 6 months of age at the start of the RSV season if they were born at 33 to 35 weeks' gestation and have 2 or more additional risk factors. Factors that increase the risk of RSV infection include

  - Exposure to environmental air pollutants
  - Congenital abnormalities of the airways
  - Severe neuromuscular disease
  - Day care attendance
  - School-aged siblings

In general, routine immunizations are delayed if a baby becomes sick, develops an infection, or is receiving a course of steroids. If illness or steroid use are not factors, any baby who has reached 8 weeks postnatal age can be given the immunizations listed below.

- **Diphtheria, tetanus, acellular pertussis (DTaP) vaccine** is given at the usual dose of 0.5 mL (contraindications to pertussis are the same in preterm as in term infants). Do *not* decrease the dose of DTaP or increase the interval between immunizations in infants requiring continuing care because these changes may not allow the baby to mount a significant antibody response.

In general, vaccine-related side effects are no more common in preterm infants than in term infants, although there are some reports of increased apnea and bradycardia spells as well as increased need for oxygen.

- **Haemophilus b conjugate vaccine** should be given in the usual dose of 0.5 mL, intramuscularly.

- **Enhanced inactivated poliovirus vaccine (IPV)** should be given in the usual dose of 0.5 mL, subcutaneously in mid-lateral thigh.

- **Pneumococcal vaccine** should be given in the usual dose of 0.5 mL, intramuscularly.

G. Screening Hearing

1. Which Babies Should Have Their Hearing Screened?

In many centers, the hearing of all infants hospitalized in intensive care units is evaluated prior to discharge. The following factors place infants at risk for hearing loss:

- Birth weight less than 1,500 g (3 lb, 5 oz)
- Any of the congenital TORCH infections
- Severe perinatal compromise
- Exposure to ototoxic medication(s)
- Bacterial meningitis
- Severe hyperbilirubinemia
- Family history of childhood hearing impairment
- Malformations that involve the head or neck
- Stigmata or other findings associated with a syndrome known to include hearing impairment

2. When and How Should Hearing Screening Be Done?

Hearing should be evaluated before discharge or by 3 months of age for all babies.

Initial screening should include behavioral or electrophysiologic response to sound, using instruments designed for newborns. If results of the initial screening are equivocal, the baby should be referred for formal diagnostic testing. All babies should continue to have routine hearing tests at well-baby examinations.

H. Screening for Retinopathy of Prematurity (ROP)

Recent development of peripheral retinal ablative therapy using laser photocoagulation and the results of large studies have redefined treatment recommendations to reduce the incidence of ROP*.

---

* American Academy of Pediatrics Section on Ophthalmology, American Academy of Ophthalmology, American Association for Pediatric Ophthalmology and Strabismus. Screening examination of premature infants for retinopathy of prematurity. *Pediatrics*. 2006;117:572–576. See also the erratum (*Pediatrics*. 2006;118:1324).

1. Which Babies Need Examinations for ROP?

   In general, the following babies should have a dilated funduscopic examination by an ophthalmologist with experience in ROP:

   - Any baby born at 30 weeks' gestation or less or with birth weight less than 1,500 g

   - Any baby with a birth weight between 1,500 and 2,000 g, but with an unstable clinical course and believed to be at high risk for ROP

2. When and How Should ROP Screening Be Done?

   Timing of the first examination depends on the baby's gestational age at birth. The initial examination may have been done at the regional medical center before the baby was discharged. First examinations should be performed on babies born at

   - 22 to 27 weeks' gestation when they reach 31 weeks' postmenstrual age

   - 28 to 32 weeks' gestation when they reach 4 weeks' chronologic age

   The timing of follow-up examinations is dictated by the findings of the first examination. If both retinas are fully vascularized at the time of the first examination, additional examinations may not be needed. If the retinas are not fully vascularized, repeat examinations are indicated, even if there is no initial evidence of ROP.

   The examining ophthalmologist will recommend follow-up examinations based on the initial retinal findings. If the retina is not fully vascularized, follow-up examinations will be recommended at intervals ranging from less than 1 week to as long as 3 weeks. The ophthalmologist will also recommend when treatment is indicated.

 To minimize the risk of retinal detachment, treatment should generally be performed within 72 hours of treatable disease being identified.

   Clear communication among providers and with parents must stress that follow-up is essential to successful therapy and that, if treatment is needed, there is a critical period in which it can be carried out to prevent severe visual loss or blindness.

I. Sleep Position and Sleeping Environment

   Prior to discharge, you should begin to accustom babies to supine sleep position. This is the safest position for a baby after discharge and has been shown to reduce the risk of SIDS. Babies initially put to sleep on their stomachs may take some time to become familiar with sleeping on their backs. By the time a baby is discharged, a back (supine) sleep position should be familiar and comfortable.

201

As a further precaution against an acute life-threatening event (ALTE), soft objects such as pillows and stuffed animals, should not be in a baby's sleeping area. Teach the parents that loose or excessively soft bedding should also be avoided.

J. Assessment of Family

1. What Factors Should You Consider?

- *Common Stress Factors*

  The birth of an at-risk or sick baby may create enormous emotional and financial stresses for a family or single parent.

  Feelings of anxiety, guilt, inadequacy, and anger are common. Additionally, geographic distance often separates the baby from parents, making visiting difficult. The family, particularly the mother, may experience a sense of isolation. Young or inexperienced parents may be overwhelmed by their new responsibilities.

- *Possible Impact*

  All these factors influence the normal process of parent-infant bonding and subsequent interactions of the baby and the baby's family. Because of the increased stresses created by the birth of an at-risk or sick baby, these babies are at risk for poor growth and neglect. Close, frequent contact between the parents and their baby is important to the development of a healthy relationship.

Personnel caring for these babies must be aware of this high-risk situation. It is important to promote parent-infant attachment and to teach parenting skills, as well as to observe family interactions.

2. How Can You Assess Parent-Infant Interaction?

There are several ways to assess parental interaction with and attachment to the baby.

- Keep a record of telephone calls made by the parents.

- Keep a record of visits.

- Keep a record of caregiving activities taught to the parents, and performed successfully by them.

- Assign one nurse to be primarily responsible for communicating with the family.

- Have daily or weekly discussions, starting from the date of admission, among the nurses, physicians, and social workers concerning the progress of parent-infant attachment and family interactions, and promptly address any identified problems.

- Start assessment immediately and modify it, as necessary, as the baby's hospital course progresses. Do *not* wait until the baby is ready for discharge to assess family interactions, teaching done and needed, and the parents' ability to care for their baby.

3. What Can You Do to Promote Parent-Infant Attachment and Positive Family Interaction?

- Maintain liberal or unlimited visiting hours.

- Make time available to instruct the mother or parents in the routine care of the baby.

- Allow and encourage the parents to care for the baby as much as possible while the baby is in the hospital (change diapers; bathe, hold, and rock the baby; provide kangaroo care [if parents wish to do so]; feed the baby; and perform any special procedures the baby will need after discharge).

- Make time to answer questions.

- Praise the parents for well-performed tasks.

- Be patient with timid and inexperienced parents.

- Involve social service and request increased assistance for families with marked social, transportation, or economic problems.

- Consider involving public health agencies to aid in assessment of the home environment.

- Arrange for the mother or parents to "room in" with the baby prior to discharge.

- Request psychiatric assistance for parent(s) with marked emotional problems.

Self-Test

Now answer these questions to test yourself on the information in the last section.

B1. **True** **False** To give a supplemental feeding, you first feed the baby as much as the baby will eat, then insert a feeding tube and give the remainder of the calculated volume of feeding.

B2. Which of the following is important in weaning a baby from an incubator to a crib?

Yes	No	
___	___	Place a stocking cap on the baby's head.
___	___	Begin antibiotics.
___	___	Give the baby at least 25% more calories.
___	___	Wrap the baby in extra blankets.

B3. If a baby's head grows more rapidly than normal, the baby may be developing _____.

B4. After being weaned to a crib, a baby does not gain weight for several days in a row. List 4 possible reasons for the lack of weight gain.

1. _____

2. _____

3. _____

4. _____

B5. Babies requiring medications to treat apnea need 2 types of monitoring.

_____

_____

B6. **True** **False** Babies may not have a gag reflex even though they are 32 to 34 weeks' estimated gestational age.

B7. **True** **False** A 2,100-g (4 lb, 10 oz) baby who requires theophylline for management of apneic spells, has had no apnea for 8 consecutive days. The baby may be safely discharged home with no additional monitoring needed.

B8. A baby should be evaluated for possible hydrocephalus if the head circumference grows more than

_____ cm/week.

B9. A normal weight gain is _____ g/day.

B10. Name 2 drugs that may be used for certain babies to decrease the number of apneic spells.

_____

_____

B11. A 1,900-g (4 lb, 3 oz) baby has an apneic spell. The baby should be monitored until no apnea has occurred

for_____ consecutive days.

B12. Name at least 3 signs that indicate when a low hematocrit may be dangerous.

_____

_____

_____

B13. Name at least 3 ways to assess parental-infant bonding.

_____

_____

_____

B14. It is recommended that a baby's

- Weight be determined every _____
- Head circumference be determined every _____
- Length be determined every _____

B15. Name 3 reasons an infant who requires continuing care may become anemic.

1. _____
2. _____
3. _____

B16. Which of the following encourage parent-infant attachment?

Yes	No	
___	___	Unlimited visiting hours
___	___	Adapting care routines for parents who wish to provide kangaroo care
___	___	Many nurses caring for the infant and talking with the family
___	___	Involvement of social service in special cases
___	___	Teaching parents how to bathe and feed their baby

B17. List 2 groups of babies who should receive an eye examination.

1. _____
2. _____

B18. **True** **False** During respiratory syncytial virus season, babies in certain groups should receive palivizumab *prior* to discharge from the hospital.

B19. **True** **False** Routine immunizations with diphtheria, tetanus, acellular pertussis; enhanced inactivated poliovirus; and pneumococcal conjugate can be given at 8 weeks of age for most preterm infants, but the dose of each vaccine should be reduced from that given to healthy term babies.

B20. **True** **False** Treatment for retinopathy of prematurity should be carried out within 72 hours of a treatable condition being identified.

Check your answers with the list that follows the Recommended Routines. Correct any incorrect answers and review the appropriate section in the unit.

5. What Is Involved in Discharge of a Baby?

Preparation for discharge is an important task. Although most babies will have few, if any, major problems at the time of discharge, care must be taken to ensure that both baby and family are ready for home care to begin.

A. What Are the Criteria for Discharge?

- Baby's weight is approximately 1,800 to 2,000 g (4 lb–4 lb, 7 oz).

- Baby is gaining weight.

- Baby can maintain normal body temperature in a crib.

- Baby is eating well by nipple or breastfeeding well every 3 to 4 hours.

- Baby has been
  - Apnea-free 7 to 8 consecutive days (on no medication)
  OR
  - Apnea-free on medication and you have detailed plans for careful follow-up of drug levels
  OR
  - Discharged on a monitor and you have detailed plans for careful follow-up
  (Note: Some centers use slightly different discharge criteria for babies with apnea.)

- Baby's medical condition is stable. For example, if the baby has congestive heart failure (CHF), it is well controlled on medications.

- Baby's hematocrit is stable or not rapidly falling. No infant who has symptoms from anemia should be discharged and, in general, infants are not discharged if the hematocrit is less than 22% to 24%.

- Appropriate neonatal screening tests have been done (metabolic screening studies, eye examinations, hearing screen, etc).

- Immunizations have been given according to the baby's age and history.
  OR
- Arrangements have been made for the baby's primary care physician to see the baby soon after discharge and to give the immunizations.

- Palivizumab has been given, as appropriate, according to the baby's age, history, risk factors, and the season of the year.

- Baby's parents have demonstrated the ability to care for their baby, and the home situation is considered acceptable.

- Baby can tolerate a car seat. The AAP recommends that any infant born at less than 37 weeks' gestation be observed in a car seat, before discharge, to monitor for apnea, bradycardia, and oxygen desaturation.

In general, the duration of observation should be longer than the length of time the baby will be in the car seat during the trip from the hospital to home. If the infant does not tolerate the car seat for this duration, the baby may not be ready for discharge, or consideration should be given to using a lying-down car bed.

B. How Do You Plan for Discharge?

- Anticipate the discharge a minimum of 2 weeks before the infant goes home.

- Notify the parents of the possible discharge date. Solicit and answer their questions and concerns.

- Notify any special individuals or groups involved in the care of the child (public health department, social services, etc).

- Check the parental visiting record and home environment. If the home situation seems unacceptable/unstable, request evaluation by public health nurse and/or social service.

- If the infant requires special medications or treatments, make certain the parents understand the infant's medical condition, are able to give the medicine appropriately, and can perform any necessary treatment.

- Perform detailed, thorough physical examination.

- Document weight, length, and head circumference measurements. These will be important for outpatient follow-up care.

- Provide car seat instruction and testing, using the same seat the parents will use for the baby.

- Talk with the parents frequently, and on the day of discharge. Answer questions, explain hospital course, and help parents anticipate course the infant will follow for the next several weeks or months.

- Review immunization schedule.

- Make appointments for well-baby care.

- Arrange for a home visiting nurse to assess baby, particularly if the baby has significant medical problems or if the social situation seems unstable.

- Make appointments, as necessary, for follow-up hearing tests and/or eye examinations. Ensure clear communication with the parents and other care providers regarding follow-up eye examinations, and the critical need to keep appointments according to the schedule recommended by the examining ophthalmologist.

- Prepare information to send to the baby's follow-up and/or primary care physicians. Include history and current status of problems, growth measurements at discharge, any medications with details about measuring serum levels and need to adjust for weight, and a list of follow-up appointments.

- Reinforce the need for the infant to be seen in the regional center follow-up clinic for serial developmental evaluations, and for further monitoring of special problems (if the baby has any).

Self-Test

Now answer these questions to test yourself on the information in the last section.

C1. **True** **False** A baby who has been started on a new drug to treat an unstable medical condition can be discharged the same day.

C2. **True** **False** An asymptomatic baby with a stable hematocrit of 22% to 24% can be discharged.

C3. A baby is medically ready for discharge. However, despite repeated attempts to contact the parents, you have been unable to reach them for 2 weeks. One day they unexpectedly appear at the hospital and want to take their baby home. What would you do?

_____

_____

_____

_____

_____

C4. List at least 5 activities important in planning for discharge.

_____

_____

_____

_____

_____

C5. **True** **False** A baby weighs 1,400 g (3 lb, 1 1/2 oz), has never had an apneic spell, and is gaining weight steadily. This baby can safely be discharged home at this time.

Check your answers with the list that follows the Recommended Routines. Correct any incorrect answers and review the appropriate section in the unit.

Subsection: Babies With Special Problems

1. What Special Problems May Be Encountered in Babies Requiring Continuing Care?

Most babies referred to you will be stable preterm infants. However, some babies who recover from an initial severe illness will develop special problems requiring frequent, but not constant, attention.

For example, some babies born extremely preterm or who required assisted ventilation for treatment of severe respiratory distress syndrome, may develop lung damage. These babies can eventually recover but may require supplemental oxygen for long periods. They may have needed numerous blood gas determinations during the acute phase of the disease. At this stage of the illness, they need blood gas analyses much less often, especially if continuous pulse oximetry is used. Sudden changes are not expected, yet the babies must be monitored for this special problem as well as receive the routine care described earlier in this unit.

The following is a list of problems sometimes seen in infants recovering from acute neonatal illnesses. If you are caring for a baby with one of these problems, your regional center can give you more specific information about the cause, treatment, and prognosis of the particular problem in that particular baby.

A. Chronic Lung Disease (CLD)

Post-neonatal CLD (formerly termed bronchopulmonary dysplasia) is a form of lung disease thought to result from the combined effects of high concentrations of oxygen and trauma to the lungs produced by high airway pressures generated by respirators. Some extremely preterm babies will develop CLD, even if they did not need therapy with a ventilator or high oxygen concentration. Babies with CLD may require supplemental oxygen by nasal cannula for weeks or even months.

In general, these babies exhibit steady improvement and progressively require less oxygen to maintain a good blood oxygen level. It is important to remember, however, not to decrease supplemental oxygen too quickly because chronic low blood oxygen may cause serious, permanent damage to the heart and lung blood vessels.

Unlike adults with CLD, these babies form new, healthy lung tissue as they grow and, therefore, may eventually recover completely. If they become ill, it is usually related to the onset of pneumonia or fluid retention.

Occasionally some babies will require supplemental oxygen for such long periods that you, the regional center, and the family decide it is most reasonable that the baby be cared for at home. These are very special cases, with the baby receiving supplemental oxygen and other medications at home, and will be managed by you and the regional center together.

B. Retinopathy of Prematurity (ROP)

ROP is an eye disease of preterm babies that may result from many different factors, including oxygen therapy. The degree of visual impairment may range from slight impairment to total blindness. The likelihood and severity increases with the degree of prematurity. Once ROP has developed it must be closely followed with repeated examinations. The damage may progress to cause retinal detachment if not treated promptly, or it may resolve completely. Previous recommendations have been replaced by the AAP policy statement "Screening Examination of Premature Infants for Retinopathy of Prematurity" (*Pediatrics*. 2006;117:572–576, Erratum. *Pediatrics*. 2006;118:1324).

At-risk preterm infants need to be examined at recommended times to detect the changes of ROP and provide treatment before permanent visual loss occurs. Detailed retinal examination and classification of disease should be carried out by an ophthalmologist with experience in ROP.

Even if laser therapy is not indicated, it is important for an ophthalmologist to follow the baby so the parents will know what to expect for and from their baby. In addition, babies who have had ROP, whether or not treatment was required, are at higher risk for other visual disorders, including strabismus, amblyopia, cataract, etc. Eyeglasses may be indicated in some cases and are most beneficial when fitted at an early age.

C. Gastroesophageal Reflux

Gastroesophageal reflux occurs when stomach contents reflux into the esophagus. This disorder, apparently more common in preterm than in term babies, is being diagnosed with increasing frequency in sick and at-risk babies. It typically presents with frequent spitting or vomiting after feedings, or continual regurgitation, and may be associated with apnea and bradycardia.

Treatment regimens may include thickening feedings and use of medications. Consult with your regional center staff to establish a treatment plan specific to each particular baby.

D. Short Bowel Syndrome

Sometimes babies are born with less than the normal length of intestines. Other babies have variable lengths of intestine removed during surgery for certain types of bowel disease, such as necrotizing enterocolitis.

Sometimes these babies have ostomies. If an ostomy is present it will require special care, and parents should receive detailed instructions. Ostomies may be permanent or the bowel may be reconnected at a later date.

Babies with a decreased amount of intestine for any reason may have trouble absorbing milk or formula. They may have problems with weight gain, blood electrolyte imbalance, and/or dehydration. They usually require special formulas, frequent weight checks, and occasional checks of blood electrolytes. Blood electrolyte samples are needed more often if the volume of ostomy output or the number of stools increase.

E.   Seizures

There are many causes of seizures in the newborn period. Babies may be sent home from nurseries on anticonvulsants, such as phenobarbital.

These infants must be monitored for the recurrence of seizures, and have their anticonvulsant drug dose adjusted as they grow. Some will require determination of blood levels of their anticonvulsant medication.

They must also be observed carefully for signs of developmental delay.

F.   Hydrocephalus

Babies ill at birth will occasionally develop hydrocephalus, particularly if they were born extremely preterm and developed an intraventricular hemorrhage. These children may require the insertion of a shunt to prevent accumulation of excess cerebrospinal fluid in the brain. The shunt may malfunction and fluid pressure may build up. These babies may also get shunt infections. Babies with shunts must be monitored for change in activity and/or increase in head size, which would suggest a shunt malfunction or infection.

Babies with mild hydrocephalus but without shunts should have head circumferences and tenseness of their fontanels checked frequently. Coordinate with the regional medical center to schedule follow-up cranial ultrasound examinations.

G.   Poor Head Growth

Poor head growth is sometimes seen in babies with severe perinatal compromise. It is more likely to occur when periventricular leukomalacia has been detected by ultrasound and is associated with an increased likelihood of poor outcome.

These babies may need special services or care interventions, and their parents will need additional counseling.

H.   Parenting Problems

Preterm or sick babies frequently become the focus of emotional and financial stress for parents. Although the baby may recover satisfactorily from the acute illness, a difficult family situation may become the baby's major problem. The families of these children must be monitored carefully before these babies can safely be sent home.

I.   Congenital Heart Disease (CHD)

Babies with CHD may be cyanotic (blue) or acyanotic (pink), depending on the type of abnormalities in the formation of their hearts.

Cyanotic babies frequently require surgery early in life. They require monitoring for the level of blood oxygen, medication levels, development of acidosis, and for blue spells.

Babies with acyanotic heart disease frequently are on medications for congestive heart failure (CHF). They require monitoring for signs of CHF and may need adjustment of their medications.

2. How Do You Care for These Special Problems?

Certain routines of monitoring and treatment should be carried out for these babies. Use the following guidelines, but do not hesitate to call the regional center if you have questions or if the baby appears to be worsening.

Note that the intervals suggested for monitoring are intended for stable babies. An unstable baby may need more frequent monitoring.

Knowledge of the best treatment for these conditions changes rapidly.

Frequent communication with your regional medical center staff is important if you are caring for a baby with a special problem.

Self-Test

Now answer these questions to test yourself on the information in the last section.

D1. Name 2 types of congenital heart disease.

_____

_____

D2. **True** **False** A baby with seizures appears normal at the time of discharge. In spite of this, the child should be assessed later for the appearance of developmental delay.

D3. Babies with hydrocephalus may require insertion of a _____

to prevent accumulation of excess cerebrospinal fluid.

D4. **True** **False** Babies who require supplemental oxygen for months generally recover and can be discharged from the hospital.

D5. **True** **False** Visual impairment from retinopathy of prematurity may range from slight impairment to total blindness.

D6. Babies with cyanotic congenital heart disease may require monitoring for

1. _____

2. _____

3. _____

4. _____

D7. Two major problems with shunts used to treat hydrocephalus are _____ and

_____ .

D8. When babies with chronic lung disease become ill it is usually with _____ or

_____ .

D9. Babies with acyanotic congenital heart disease frequently are on medications for

_____

D10. The dose of anticonvulsant drugs should be adjusted according to the
   A. Length of the baby
   B. Weight of the baby
   C. Head circumference of the baby

Check your answers with the list that follows the Recommended Routines. Correct any incorrect answers and review the appropriate section in the unit.

Monitoring and Treatment Guidelines for Babies With Special Problems

A. Chronic Lung Disease (CLD) (formerly termed bronchopulmonary dysplasia)

Monitoring	Reason for Monitoring	Abnormality	Action
Weight (every day)	Babies with CLD may retain fluid in their lungs and may have right heart failure.	• Rapid increase in weight gain	• Decrease baby's fluid intake. • Increase or begin diuretics.
	Babies with CLD require more energy to breathe. Therefore, they may require more than the normal number of calories to breathe and grow.	• Lack of weight gain	• Review concentration of calories in formula or breast milk supplements. • Check the baby's blood oxygen level. Babies with chronically low blood oxygen will not gain weight well.
Medications	Babies with CLD frequently are on several medications. These medications may require frequent adjustment. Some medications are routinely tapered, while others are gradually increased as the baby grows.	• Worsening arterial blood gases • Increased weight gain	• Increase the dose appropriate for the weight.
• Dexamethasone	This medication is no longer recommended, except for babies with severe CLD.	• Following a course of Decadron, lung disease may worsen.	• If you receive a baby on a tapering dosage regimen of Decadron, consult regional center staff. • Monitor oxygen saturation, especially as the medication is being tapered.
• Aminophylline	Babies with CLD often have bronchospasm. Aminophylline is frequently used as a bronchodilator for these babies. Dose (after loading dose): 1.5–3.0 mg/kg/dose, q6–8h, depending on baby's age	• Increased wheezing (too little drug) • Tachycardia 180 (too much drug)	• Monitor level and adjust dose (keep approximately 10–12 mcg/mL). May need to increase dose based on serum level. • Many need to decrease or hold dose based on serum level.
• Albuterol	Nebulized albuterol is frequently used to decrease bronchospasm in babies with CLD. Dose: 0.1–0.5 mg/kg/dose, every 4–6 hours	• Increased wheezing (too little drug) • Tachycardia 180 (too much drug)	• Give STAT dose; monitor heart rate. • May need to hold dose and increase interval between doses.
• Spironolactone (Aldactone)	Dose: 1–3 mg/kg/dose every 24h, given orally		
• Furosemide (Lasix) • Chlorothiazide	Dose: 1–4 mg/kg/day divided into 3–4 doses Dose: 10–20 mg/kg/dose every 12–24 hours, given orally	• Electrolyte abnormalities (hypochloremic alkalosis from chloride loss) • Osteopenia and kidney stones from serum calcium loss	• Monitor serum electrolytes. • Try to wean off medication as lung disease improves. • Consider adding potassium chloride (KCl) to feedings.

A. Chronic Lung Disease (CLD) (formerly termed bronchopulmonary dysplasia), continued

Monitoring	Reason for Monitoring	Abnormality	Action
Hematocrit (every week)	Babies with CLD may become worse if they become anemic.	• Hematocrit <35% for babies still requiring oxygen therapy	• Look for cause of anemia. • Treat cause of anemia. • Consider transfusion if oxygen requirements are high and baby is not improving.
Electrolytes (every week)	Diuretics may cause abnormalities in serum sodium (Na^+), potassium (K^+), chloride (Cl^-), and/or calcium (Ca^+). Low chloride has been associated with poor growth and poor outcome. High calcium has been associated with renal calculi.	• Decreased Na^+, K^+, Cl^-	• Increase Na^+, K^+, Cl^- in diet. • However, consider that a decrease in serum Na^+ in face of increased weight may indicate excess fluid retention, in which case NaCl therapy would be contraindicated. • Consider decreasing dose of furosemide and/or adding spironolactone.
	CLD may lead to fluid overload with a dilutional decrease of serum Na^+.	• Decreased Na^+	• Assess for weight gain. Restrict fluids, increase diuretics.
Chest x-ray	Babies with CLD frequently develop pneumonia.	• Pneumonia (always compare with prior baseline x-ray)	• Consider antibiotics. • Provide chest physical therapy.
Electrocardiogram or Echocardiogram	CLD may lead to right ventricular hypertrophy.	• Worsening right ventricular hypertrophy (RVH)	• Make certain baby's PaO_2 is 60 mm Hg or higher and/or oxygen saturation is 90%–94% during sleep and all activities. • Make certain baby is on adequate doses of diuretics. • Consult regional center if there is worsening RVH; CLD may be inadequately treated.
Heart rate monitoring	Any hospitalized baby requiring supplemental oxygen should have continuous electronic heart rate monitoring. The heart rate may decrease if the baby's PaO_2 decreases.	• Bradycardia	• Administer oxygen. • Assess for increased secretions, blocked airway. • Assess for infection.
Physical findings Note: *Sustained decrease in respiratory rate is a good indicator of improvement.*	Babies with CLD frequently have reactive airways and demonstrate marked bronchospasm (wheezing). Often these babies require bronchodilators. Bronchospasm can also result from chronic hypoxia.	• Increased wheezing	• Assess arterial blood gas and/or oxygen saturation. • Assess bronchodilator level/dose and diuretic dose. • Consider STAT dose of an inhaled bronchodilator. • Assess for pneumonia.
	Rales may be due to infection, or fluid retention in the lungs. Babies with CLD may also have hepatosplenomegaly from right heart failure.	• Increased rales and increased hepatosplenomegaly	• Assess arterial blood gas or oxygen saturation. • Assess diuretic dose. • Assess for pneumonia.
	Babies with CLD may have excess secretions that, if not removed, predispose the baby to pneumonia.	• Excess secretions, signs of pneumonia	• Increase frequency of chest physical therapy. Give at least twice a day. • Assess for pneumonia.

A. Chronic Lung Disease (CLD) (formerly termed bronchopulmonary dysplasia), continued

Monitoring	Reason for Monitoring	Abnormality	Action
Supplemental inspired oxygen concentration (FiO_2)	As the baby improves, you will be able to lower the FiO_2 required to maintain a PaO_2 of approximately 60 mm Hg and an oxygen saturation of 90%–94%.		
	Any FiO_2 greater than that necessary to maintain a PaO_2 of 60 mm Hg (or oxygen saturation of 90%–94%) may be unnecessarily damaging to the lungs of babies with chronic disease.	• Persistently high FiO_2	• Monitor arterial blood gases or oxygen saturation. • Decrease FiO_2 for consistent PaO_2 >70 mm Hg or oxygen saturation >94%.
	Too low an FiO_2 may cause a low PaO_2, increased bronchospasm, decreased blood flow to the lungs, and may also inhibit the baby's growth.	• Cyanosis, increased bronchospasm, tachypnea, or wheezing	• Monitor arterial blood gases or oxygen saturation. • Increase FiO_2 for consistent PaO_2 <60 mm Hg or oxygen saturation <90%.
Blood gas	Initially, blood gases are monitored frequently on sick babies; but monitoring frequency decreases as the baby grows older and more stable. Generally, capillary blood gases 1–2 times/week with continuous pulse oximetry provide adequate monitoring.		
• Oxygen	PaO_2 should be kept approximately 60 mm Hg. Oxygen saturation, during all activities (feeding, sleeping), should be kept at 90%–94%.	• PaO_2 below 60 mm Hg or oxygen saturation below 90%	• Increase supplemental oxygen. • Look for cause of decreased PaO_2 (pneumonia, increased secretions, worsening right heart failure). • Assess for bronchospasm.
• Carbon dioxide	Carbon dioxide is usually increased in CLD. • If CO_2 is getting progressively higher, the baby's condition is worsening. • If the CO_2 is decreasing, the baby is improving.	• Increased $PaCO_2$ over baseline value	• Assess for pneumonia. • Obtain chest x-ray. • Suction secretions.
• pH	pH is usually normal in these babies. If it is increased or decreased, the baby may be worsening or improving.	• Decrease in pH	• Assess for bronchospasm. • Assess for pneumonia. • Obtain chest x-ray. • Suction secretions.

B. Retinopathy of Prematurity (ROP) (formerly termed retrolental fibroplasia)

Monitoring	Reason for Monitoring	Abnormality	Action
Evaluation by ophthalmologist	Examine babies born at ≤30 weeks' gestation or with birth weight <1,500 g and babies with a birth weight between 1,500–2,000 g, but with an unstable clinical course and believed to be at high risk for ROP. If the retinas are not fully vascularized, repeat exams are indicated by gestational age and retinal status, even if there was no initial evidence of ROP. Dilated funduscopic exam should be done by an ophthalmologist with experience in ROP.		• Laser coagulation therapy may be helpful. If needed, it should be performed within 72 hours of a treatable condition being identified. • Contact your regional center staff for information concerning management and referral. • Have corrective eyeglasses (if prescribed) fitted early.
Family's understanding of the disease and interaction with their baby	Families may have difficulty accepting the fact that their baby may have significant visual impairment. They may have unrealistic expectations for the baby's development (either too pessimistic or too optimistic).	• Denial by the family of the baby's condition	Counsel family that • Keeping exam, treatment, and follow-up appointments is essential for optimal preservation of sight. • The condition will not go away; anger is normal. • Developmental milestones may be different for their baby than for a baby with normal sight. • Contact nearby agencies for the blind or visually impaired to acquaint family with local resources.

C. Gastroesophageal Reflux (GER)

Monitoring	Reason for Monitoring	Abnormality	Action
Weight	Babies with GER may regurgitate so much that they do not gain weight satisfactorily.	• Lack of weight gain	• Adjust medications.
Medications	Babies with GER often are on medications to inhibit gastric acid secretion (acid stomach contents can cause inflammation of the esophagus) and sometimes are on medications to improve gastric emptying and gastrointestinal motility.		
• Ranitidine or famotidine	Dose: 2 mg/kg, orally, every 8 hours	• Failure to gain weight	• Adjust dose for weight. • Consult regional center staff.
• Metoclopramide	Dose: 0.033–0.1 mg/kg, orally or slow IV push, every 8 hours	• Continued regurgitation • Failure to gain weight	• Adjust dose for weight. • Consult regional center staff; use in GER is controversial.

D. Short Bowel Syndrome

Monitoring	Reason for Monitoring	Abnormality	Action
Weight (every day)	An increase in weight is a sign of adequate intake and absorption. A decrease in weight is a sign of malabsorption.	• Decrease in weight	• Assess caloric intake. • Assess number of stools or volume of ostomy output, stool pH, electrolytes, and blood urea nitrogen (BUN).
	Babies who have an increased number of stools or increased ostomy output are malabsorbing their formula.	• Increase in output	• Assess for malabsorption of carbohydrates by checking pH of the stool. pH <6 suggests carbohydrate malabsorption. • Put baby on 1/2-strength formula or clear liquids temporarily.
Stool pH	Assess if poor weight gain or increase in stools or ostomy output. An acid pH means there is poor absorption of sugar.	• Acid pH (6)	• Decrease intake of sugar or consider changing to non-lactose formula.
Electrolytes and BUN	Babies with increased fluid losses through the intestine may develop electrolyte abnormalities.	• Decreased Na^+, K^+ • Decreased K^+ • Increased BUN	• Increase Na^+ in diet. • Increase K^+ in diet. • Assess for signs of dehydration and consider administration of IV fluids.
Family understanding of condition	Family must be educated regarding ostomy care, or care of buttocks, and taught warning signs such as increase in stools or ostomy output.	• Lack of instruction • Lack of interest	• Teach family importance of their care and observations. • Observe family provide all details of care.

E. Seizures

Monitoring	Reason for Monitoring	Abnormality	Action
Anticonvulsant drug(s)	As the baby grows and gains weight the anticonvulsant dose will need to be increased. After a loading dose to achieve suppression of seizures, use a maintenance dose of 3.5–5 mg/kg/day of phenobarbital. Measure serum levels periodically. Adjust dose as necessary to keep a serum level of 20–30 mcg/mL.	• Increase in seizure activity	• Adjust dose of anticonvulsant. • Consult regional center staff.

F. Hydrocephalus

Monitoring	Reason for Monitoring	Abnormality	Action
Head circumference (daily)	Worsening hydrocephalus or a malfunctioning shunt will cause head circumference to increase.	Head circumference increase >1.25 cm/week or 0.25 cm/day, over several days	• Obtain cranial ultrasound. • Consult regional center staff.
Signs of infection	Babies with shunts in place may develop infections around or within the shunt.	• Irritability • Lethargy • Vomiting • Fever • Tense fontanel	• Obtain blood cultures, CBC, etc. • Consult regional center staff.

G. Poor Head Growth

Monitoring	Reason for Monitoring	Abnormality	Action
Head circumference (weekly)	Provide continued surveillance of babies with severe perinatal compromise.	Head circumference does not increase at least 0.5 cm/week for several weeks	• Assess caloric intake and weight gain. • Monitor developmental progress. • Obtain cranial ultrasound. • Discuss concerns with family. • Consult regional center staff.

H. Poor Parental-Infant Attachment

Monitoring	Reason for Monitoring	Abnormality	Action
Number of visits/phone calls	Sick or preterm babies are more frequently neglected than healthy, term infants.	• Few visits • Few phone calls	• Make time to listen to parents, counsel parents, and teach parenting and caregiving skills.
Interaction among family members	Preterm infants are also more often born to mothers who are • Young • Poor • Substance users	• Excessive friction among family members	• Involve your hospital's social service department. • Consult public health department. • Consult psychiatry if family problems are severe.
Parenting skills		• Poor parenting skills	• Detain the baby until family/social problems are resolved or situation is stable enough for baby to be discharged.
Readiness of home		• No readiness in the home for the baby	• Arrange frequent follow-up by visiting nurse and follow-up visits with physician.

I. Congenital Heart Disease (CHD)

Monitoring	Reason for Monitoring	Abnormality	Action
Heart rate	Worsening congestive heart failure (CHF) or hypoxia will affect heart rate.	• Increase in heart rate • Decrease in heart rate	• Assess for CHF. • Assess for hypoxia.
Weight (every day)	Worsening CHF will result in fluid retention and excessive weight gain.	• Weight gain >20–30 g/day • Decrease in weight	• Assess for increasing CHF (increased rales, increased hepatosplenomegaly). • Consider an increase in diuretic dose. • Assess for inadequate caloric intake.
Hematocrit (every 3–4 days)	A low hematocrit may cause CHF. High hematocrit may mean chronically worse hypoxia in a cyanotic baby.	• <30% • >60%	• Assess cause for anemia. • Assess for increasing CHF. • Consult regional center staff.
Medications	Babies with heart disease may be on medications that will need to be increased with growth and weight gain.		
Digoxin	Heart contractility and some arrhythmias are improved with digoxin. Excessive digoxin causes arrhythmias.	• Worsening CHF • Arrhythmias	• Adjust dosage appropriate for weight. Consider monitoring blood levels. • Obtain electrocardiogram. • Measure blood level.
Diuretics	Diuretics help prevent fluid retention resulting from CHF.	• Worsening CHF	• Increase dose appropriate for weight.
Electrolytes (every week)	Diuretics may cause excessive Na^+, K^+, Cl^-, and/or calcium loss.	• Decrease in Na^+ • Decrease in K^+ • Decrease in Cl^- • Hypercalciuria	• Carefully increase Na^+ supplement, but consider that a decrease in serum Na^+ in face of increased weight may indicate worsening CHF. • Increase K^+ supplement. • Increase Cl^- supplement (usually as KCl) or decrease diuretic dose. • Monitor for renal calculi with urinalysis and possible renal ultrasound.

I. Congenital Heart Disease (CHD), continued

Monitoring	Reason for Monitoring	Abnormality	Action
Chest x-ray	Observe for signs of CHF or pneumonia.	• Lung infiltrates and/or enlarging heart size	• Increase diuretics. • Consider antibiotics.
Electrocardiogram or Echocardiogram	Babies with heart disease may develop worsening right or left ventricular hypertrophy or demonstrate arrhythmias.	• Increasing left or right ventricular hypertrophy • Development of arrhythmias	• Consult regional center staff.
Physical exam	Worsening CHF will cause increased rales, hepatosplenomegaly, and a gallop rhythm of the heart.	• Increased rales • Increased hepatosplenomegaly • Presence of gallop	• Adjust diuretic(s) for weight. • Consult regional center staff.

Recommended Routines

All of the routines listed below are based on the principles of perinatal care presented in the unit you have just finished. They are recommended as part of routine perinatal care.

Read each routine carefully and decide whether it is standard operating procedure in your hospital. Check the appropriate blank next to each routine.

Procedure Standard in My Hospital	Needs Discussion by Our Staff	
_____	_____	1. Establish the following policies for continuing care babies:
_____	_____	• Maintain in an incubator until the baby weighs approximately 1,600 (3 lb, 81/2 oz) to 1,700 g (3 lb, 12 oz).
_____	_____	• Feed by tube feedings until the baby reaches 32 to 34 weeks' gestational age, demonstrates a gag reflex, and can coordinate sucking and breathing.
_____	_____	• Weigh daily.
_____	_____	• Measure head circumference and length weekly.
_____	_____	• Monitor for apnea until the baby
_____	_____	• Weighs 1,800 g (4 lb)
_____	_____	• Reaches a gestational age of 35 weeks
_____	_____	• Has been apnea-free for 7 to 8 consecutive days (off medication).
_____	_____	• Periodically measure the baby's hematocrit. Discharge the baby on iron-fortified formula and/or supplemental iron, unless there are contraindications.
_____	_____	• Start assessment of the home environment and begin to teach caregiving skills as soon as a baby is admitted.
_____	_____	• Record family visiting patterns and performance of caregiving skills.
_____	_____	2. Develop a predischarge checklist to review for all continuing care babies.
_____	_____	3. Develop a system for periodically communicating with the regional center staff regarding the progress of any continuing care baby who has a special problem.

These are the answers to the self-test questions. Please check them with the answers you gave and review the information in the unit wherever necessary.

A1.   1. Additional weight gain
      2. Monitoring of special problems
A2.   Any 7 of the following:
      • Temperature control
      • Feeding
      • Assessment of growth
      • Apnea monitoring
      • Monitoring for anemia
      • Assessment of family
      • Administering immunizations
      • Screening of hearing
      • Screening for retinopathy of prematurity
      • Accustoming baby to supine (back) sleep position
      • Late head ultrasound
A3.   1. Weight
      2. Head circumference
      3. Length
A4.   Apnea, 1,800 g, 35 weeks, 7 to 8 days
A5.   True

B1.   False   A feeding tube should not be inserted during or shortly after a feeding. Doing so may cause the baby to vomit, and thus increase the risk that the baby will aspirate some of the feeding.
B2.   Yes   No
      _x_   ___   Place a stocking cap on the baby's head.
      ___   _x_   Begin antibiotics.
      ___   _x_   Give the baby at least 25% more calories.
      _x_   ___   Wrap the baby in extra blankets.
B3.   Hydrocephalus
B4.   1. Baby is cold
      2. Inadequate caloric intake
      3. Baby is acidotic
      4. Baby is infected (septic)
B5.   Continuous electronic heart and respiratory rate monitoring
      Checking blood level of the medication
B6.   True
B7.   False   Prior to discharge, babies should be apnea-free for 7 to 8 consecutive days after the medications have been stopped and baby's blood tested and shown to be drug-free (except in very rare circumstances when home monitoring may be used and careful follow-up is ensured).
B8.   1.25 cm/week
B9.   20 to 30 g/day
B10. Theophylline and caffeine
B11. 7 to 8 consecutive days
B12. Any 3 of the following:
      • Sustained heart rate faster than 160 beats per minute
      • Sustained respiratory rate faster than 60 breaths per minute
      • Onset or increase in apneic spells
      • Poor feeding and poor weight gain
B13. Any 3 of the following ways:
      • Record telephone calls and visits made by the parents.

224

- Record caretaking activities taught to parents and performed by them.
- Assign 1 nurse to be the primary nurse communicating with the family.
- Have regular, frequent discussions among the nurses, doctors, and social workers concerning parent-baby attachment and family interactions.
- Start assessment early, so there is time to address any problems or provide adequate teaching before the baby is ready for discharge to home.

B14. *Weight:* daily

Head circumference: weekly

Length: weekly

B15. 1. Blood taken for laboratory tests
2. Iron deficiency
3. Normal drop in hemoglobin and hematocrit that occurs in all babies in the weeks following birth

B16. Yes   No

  x   Unlimited visiting hours

  x   Adapting care routines for parent who wish to provide kangaroo care

        x   Many nurses caring for the infant and talking with the family

  x   Involvement of social service in special cases

  x   Teaching the parents to bathe and feed their baby

B17. 1. Any baby born at 30 weeks' gestation or less or with birth weight 1,500 g or less
2. Any baby with a birth weight 1,500 g to 2,000 g with unstable course and thought to be at high risk for retinopathy of prematurity

B18. True

B19. False   Diphtheria, tetanus, acellular pertussis; haemophilus influenzae Type b conjugate; enhanced inactivated poliovirus; and pneumococcal conjugate vaccines should each be given in the usual dose of 0.5 mL, for preterm and term babies.

B20. True

C1. False   Babies requiring medication should have their conditions stabilized and their response to any new medication assessed before being discharged.

C2. True   However, babies with signs of anemia should *not* be discharged.

C3. Evaluate the parents' readiness and ability to care for their baby at home.
- Observe the parents taking care of their baby (feeding, bathing, diapering, etc). Encourage the parents to visit for several hours and/or days. Assist them in making these arrangements.
- Ask the parents what preparations they have made at home for the baby.
- Determine a system for medical follow-up for the baby.
- Find out what questions and/or misunderstandings the parents have about their baby. Provide them with the correct information.
- Contact social service, public health department, etc, if additional assistance or follow-up care is needed.

C4. Any 5 of the following:
- Plan ahead.
- Determine if the baby is medically ready for discharge.
- Review parental visiting record and interaction with baby.
- Assess the parents' ability to care for their baby. Solicit and answer their questions and concerns.
- Assess parents' ability to give medications and/or provide special care measures, if the baby needs any.
- Notify any special individuals or groups involved in the baby's care; make appointments for well baby care, and for any special follow-up examinations that may be needed.
- Determine if preparations have been made in the home for the baby. Assess home environment.
- Determine what medical and/or social service follow-up will be needed and how this will be done.

- Document weight, length, head circumference.
- Perform detailed physical examination. Prepare information to send to the baby's follow-up and primary care physicians.
- Review immunizations; make appointments, as necessary, for follow-up hearing and eye examinations.
- Provide car seat testing and use instructions.

C5. False   Preterm babies are at risk for apneic spells until they reach a weight of 1,800 g or more and a gestational age of 35 weeks or more.

D1. Cyanotic (babies are blue), acyanotic (babies are pink)
D2. True
D3. Shunt
D4. True
D5. True
D6. 1. Arterial oxygen concentration
     2. Blood level of drugs used to treat their condition
     3. Development of acidosis
     4. "Blue spells" or times when the baby becomes extremely cyanotic
D7. Shunt malfunction or blockage and infection
D8. Pneumonia or fluid retention
D9. Congestive heart failure, medications such as digoxin and diuretics
D10. B. Weight of the baby

Unit 8 Posttest

Without referring back to the information in the unit, please answer the following questions. Select the *one best* answer to each question (unless otherwise instructed). Record your answers on the answer sheet that is the last page in this book *and* on the test.

1. Which of the following should you do when a stable preterm baby reaches a weight of 1,600 to 1,700 g (3 lb, 81/2 oz–3 lb, 12 oz)?

   A. Discharge the baby to home.
   B. Put a cap on the baby, wrap the baby in blankets, and turn off the heat in the incubator.
   C. Discontinue heart rate and respiratory monitoring.
   D. Put the baby in a crib and maintain the nursery temperature at 22.2°C (72°F).

2. Which of the following is the best management of a 2,100-g (4 lb, 10 oz) baby who has had an apneic spell but is otherwise well?

   A. Monitor the baby in the hospital until apnea-free for 7 to 8 days and then discharge.
   B. Start the baby on 10 mg/kg/day of theophylline and discharge home.
   C. Restrict feeding by mouth and evaluate for hydrocephalus.
   D. Discharge home with instructions to parents to observe baby frequently for further apnea.

3. A 1,600-g (3 lb, 8 oz) 6-week-old preterm baby has a hematocrit of 23%. This degree of anemia requires a blood transfusion when the

   A. Baby's heart rate increases to 160 beats per minute with crying.
   B. Baby has a decreased number of stools.
   C. Baby gains weight at a rate of 30 to 40 g/day.
   D. Baby has an increased number of severe apneic spells.

4. Which of the following actions are appropriate in assessing poor weight gain in a 3-week-old, 1,800-g (4 lb) preterm infant?

Yes	No	
___	___	Assess caloric intake.
___	___	Assess baby's temperature.
___	___	Assess baby's blood pH.
___	___	Consider evaluation for infection.

5. **True False** A stable preterm baby who weighs 1,600 g (3 lb, 8 1/2 oz) and has never had an apneic spell should have continuous electronic monitoring for apnea.

6. **True False** Before any preterm baby is discharged, it is important that the parents understand the baby will have delayed development and require special education.

7. **True False** Once an infant's seizures are controlled on a certain drug dose, the dosage does not need to be changed as the baby grows.

8. **True False** When alternating tube feedings and nipple feedings for a preterm baby, the feeding tube is inserted immediately after a nipple feeding.

9. **True False** The experience of having a sick preterm baby strengthens family ties and encourages the normal process of maternal-infant bonding.

10. **True False** After a preterm baby, stable and growing well, is discharged from the nursery, it is safe to assume that anemia will not be a problem.

11. **True False** A preterm baby who receives no greater than 25% inspired oxygen concentration can develop retinopathy of prematurity.

12. **True False** Once a baby develops chronic lung disease, it is unlikely the baby will live beyond infancy.

13. A 6-week-old baby has been hospitalized since birth but will be ready for discharge in the next several days. All of the following should be done *except*

    A. Check parental visiting records.
    B. Record baby's weight, length, and head circumference.
    C. Vaccinate the baby against measles.
    D. Make an appointment for a well-baby follow-up visit.

14. A baby with congenital heart disease was transferred back from the regional center to your nursery. He has just had a severe blue spell. Which of the following is the best action to take?

    A. Administer oxygen and observe the baby for recurrence of a blue spell.
    B. Administer oxygen, assess the baby for metabolic acidosis, and call the regional center.
    C. Leave the baby alone and call the regional center.
    D. Administer oxygen, digoxin, phenobarbital, and call the regional center.

15. A baby with necrotizing enterocolitis had a damaged portion of her small bowel removed and now requires a special formula. She weighs 2,200 g (4 lb, 13 oz) and is pink and vigorous but has lost weight for 2 days and has an increased number of stools. What should you do?

Yes	No	
___	___	Determine the pH of her stools.
___	___	Check her blood electrolytes.
___	___	Feed her by nasogastric or orogastric tube.
___	___	Keep her in an incubator.
___	___	Administer intravenous antibiotics.

16. The head circumference of a stable preterm infant in your nursery increased by 2.5 cm/week for 2 weeks in a row. Which of the following should you do?

    A. Prepare for emergency insertion of a shunt.
    B. Restrict the baby's fluids.
    C. Perform a thorough physical examination on the baby and refer the baby to the regional center for evaluation of hydrocephalus.
    D. Continue to measure the head circumference weekly for 2 more weeks.

17. Which of the following babies is at *highest* risk for developing chronic lung disease?

    A. 32-week appropriate for gestational age baby who required supplemental oxygen via an oxyhood for 8 days
    B. 42-week small for gestational age baby who required prolonged resuscitation with 100% oxygen at birth
    C. 36-week appropriate for gestational age baby who had a pneumothorax and needed 5 days of oxygen via an oxyhood
    D. 36-week appropriate for gestational age baby who required oxygen therapy and mechanical ventilation for 2 weeks

For each question, please make sure you have marked your answer on the test and on the answer sheet (last page in book). The test is for you; the answer sheet will need to be turned in for continuing education credit.

PCEP

Perinatal Continuing Education Program

Answer Key
Book III: Specialized Newborn Care

Unit 1: Review: Is the Baby Sick? Identifying and Caring for Sick and At-Risk Infants

Pretest

1. A. Yes No
- ___ _x_ Supplemental oxygen
- _x_ ___ Gestational age and size exam
- _x_ ___ Blood glucose screening test
- ___ _x_ Start IV, give glucose
- _x_ ___ Frequent vital signs

1. B. Yes No
- ___ _x_ SGA
- _x_ ___ Preterm
- _x_ ___ LGA
- ___ _x_ Post-term

1. C. Yes No
- _x_ ___ Hypoglycemia
- ___ _x_ Diarrhea
- ___ _x_ Meconium aspiration
- _x_ ___ RDS
- ___ _x_ Neonatal diabetes

1. D. Yes No
- _x_ ___ Start oral feeding
- ___ _x_ Antibiotics
- ___ _x_ Phototherapy lights
- _x_ ___ Repeat blood glucose screening test
- ___ _x_ Oxygen
- ___ _x_ Healthy, full term

2. A. Do Sev. Not
Immed. Min. Indicated
- ___ _x_ ___ Blood glucose screening test
- ___ ___ _x_ Epinephrine
- ___ _x_ ___ Connect oximeter
- _x_ ___ ___ Bag-and-mask ventilation
- ___ ___ _x_ Stimulate with water
- ___ _x_ ___ Hematocrit
- ___ _x_ ___ Blood pressure
- ___ _x_ ___ Blood gas
- ___ _x_ ___ Temperature

2. B. Yes No
- _x_ ___ Common problem
- _x_ ___ Sepsis
- _x_ ___ Hypoglycemia
- _x_ ___ Aspirated formula
- ___ _x_ Blood oxygen too high

Posttest

1. A. Yes No
- _x_ ___ Temperature
- _x_ ___ Blood pressure
- _x_ ___ Hematocrit
- _x_ ___ Blood glucose screening test
- _x_ ___ Oxygen
- _x_ ___ Oximeter

1. B. Yes No
- _x_ ___ Normal saline IV bolus, slowly
- ___ _x_ Normal saline IV bolus, quickly
- ___ _x_ Early feeding
- _x_ ___ Arterial blood gas
- _x_ ___ Chest x-ray
- _x_ ___ Cardiorespiratory monitor

1. C. Yes No
- _x_ ___ Type and cross-match blood
- _x_ ___ IV sodium bicarbonate
- _x_ ___ IV glucose
- ___ _x_ Bath
- _x_ ___ Increase oxygen
- _x_ ___ Insert UAC

1. D. C

2. A. Yes No
- _x_ ___ Chest compressions
- ___ _x_ Antibiotics
- ___ _x_ Restrict oxygen
- _x_ ___ Ventilation

2. B. Yes No
- _x_ ___ Blood pH
- _x_ ___ Blood glucose screening test
- ___ _x_ Bathe baby
- _x_ ___ Hematocrit
- _x_ ___ Blood pressure
- ___ _x_ Physical and gest. age exam
- _x_ ___ Temperature

2. C. Yes No
- _x_ ___ Reintubate, assist ventilation
- ___ _x_ IV sodium bicarbonate
- ___ _x_ Chest compressions
- _x_ ___ Portable x-ray
- ___ _x_ Blood transfusion
- ___ _x_ Glucose, slow IV push

229

Unit 2: Preparation for Neonatal Transport

Pretest

1. A. Yes No
   - x ___ Oxygen
   - ___ x Send to x-ray
   - ___ x Tube feeding
   - x ___ Arterial blood gas
   - x ___ Blood glucose test screening test
   - x ___ Pulse oximeter

1. B. C

2. Yes No
   - x ___ Peripheral IV
   - ___ x Blood culture
   - x ___ Blood glucose screening test
   - x ___ Blood pressure
   - ___ x Electrocardiogram

3. D

4. Yes No
   - ___ x Oxygen
   - x ___ Blood glucose screening test
   - ___ x Chest x-ray
   - ___ x Insert UAC
   - x ___ Peripheral IV
   - ___ x Feed by mouth

5. Yes No
   - x ___ Sodium bicarbonate
   - ___ x Bag and mask
   - ___ x Intubate and ventilate
   - x ___ Increase oxygen

6. Yes No
   - ___ x Antibiotics, then blood culture
   - x ___ Insert IV
   - x ___ Hematocrit
   - x ___ Blood glucose screening test
   - ___ x Tube feeding
   - x ___ Blood gas
   - ___ x Weigh baby

7. Yes No
   - x ___ Blood pressure
   - x ___ Repeat blood glucose screening test
   - ___ x Oxygen
   - ___ x Chest x-ray

8. False

Posttest

1. C
2. True
3. Yes No
   - x ___ Glucose
   - x ___ Calcium
   - x ___ Lumbar puncture
4. Yes No
   - x ___ Crossmatch blood
   - ___ x Serum calcium
   - ___ x Phenobarbital
   - x ___ Hematocrit
5. Yes No
   - x ___ Start IV
   - ___ x Give fluid bolus
   - x ___ Blood gas
   - x ___ Chest x-ray
   - x ___ Blood glucose screening test
   - ___ x Lumbar puncture
6. Yes No
   - ___ x Volume expander
   - ___ x Oxygen
   - x ___ Warm baby
   - x ___ Hematocrit
   - ___ x Chest x-ray
   - x ___ Begin IV
   - ___ x Feed by mouth
   - ___ x Bathe baby
7. Yes No
   - ___ x Skull x-ray
   - x ___ Blood gas
   - x ___ Oxygen
   - ___ x Blood volume expander
   - x ___ Breath sounds
   - x ___ Chest x-ray
8. A. Yes No
   - x ___ Oxyhood
   - ___ x Send to x-ray
   - ___ x Tube feedings
   - x ___ Arterial blood gas
   - x ___ Blood glucose screening test
8. B. D

Unit 3: Direct Blood Pressure Monitoring

Pretest

1. C
2. True
3. True
4. False
5. True
6. A
7. D

Posttest

1. C
2. B
3. True
4. False
5. False
6. B
7. D

Unit 4: Exchange, Reduction, and Direct Transfusions

Pretest

1. True
2. True
3. False
4. False
5. C
6. D
7. A
8. True
9. True
10. False
11. False
12. D
13. A
14. B

Posttest

1. True
2. False
3. True
4. False
5. D
6. A
7. B
8. C
9. B
10. D
11. A
12. C
13. False
14. True

Unit 5: Continuous Positive Airway Pressure

Pretest

1. A
2. D
3. False
4. C
5. B
6. B

Posttest

1. True
2. False
3. D
4. C
5. B
6. C

Unit 6: Assisted Ventilation With Mechanical Ventilators

Pretest

1. E
2. B
3. A
4. B
5. D
6. C

Posttest

1. B
2. B
3. B
4. C
5. C
6. B

Unit 7: Surfactant Therapy

Pretest

1. A
2. C
3. A
4. D
5. B
6. A
7. False
8. True
9. True
10. False
11. True

Posttest

1. D
2. D
3. A
4. D
5. B
6. D
7. False
8. True
9. False
10. False

Unit 8: Continuing Care for At-Risk Infants

Pretest

1. A
2. Yes   No
   - x   ___ Social service consult
   - x   ___ Call parents
   - ___   x Begin foster home plans
3. B
4. D
5. Yes   No
   - x   ___ Head circumference weekly
   - ___   x Start phenobarbital
   - x   ___ Weigh baby daily
   - ___   x Give Imferon
   - x   ___ Hematocrit weekly
   - x   ___ Attach cardiac or respiratory monitor
6. True
7. False
8. False
9. True
10. False
11. False
12. False
13. False
14. C
15. B
16. D
17. Yes   No
   - x   ___ Blood electrolytes
   - x   ___ Urine output
   - ___   x Stool pH
   - x   ___ Hematocrit
   - x   ___ Weight gain
   - ___   x Blood calcium

Posttest

1. B
2. A
3. D
4. Yes   No
   - x   ___ Assess caloric intake
   - x   ___ Assess baby's temperature
   - x   ___ Assess baby's blood pH
   - x   ___ Evaluate for infection
5. True
6. False
7. False
8. False
9. False
10. False
11. True
12. False
13. C
14. B
15. Yes   No
   - x   ___ Stool pH
   - x   ___ Blood electrolytes
   - ___   x Feed by NG or OG tube
   - ___   x Incubator
   - ___   x Administer antibiotics
16. C
17. D

Index

Evaluation Form
Book III: Specialized Newborn Care

Note: Completion of this form, as well as the unit pretests and posttests, is required for continuing education credit.

Date: _____

Your Name: _____   Your Hospital: _____

Work Area: Maternal/Fetal Care _____   Maternal/Fetal and Newborn Care _____

Maternal/Newborn Care _____   Newborn Care _____   Neonatal Intensive Care _____

Discipline: Physician ___   RN ___   LPN ___   AIDE ___   CNM ___   NP ___   RRT ___   Other ____

For each scale, place an "X" on the line at the point which best describes how you feel.

1. Were the objectives listed on page 2 of each unit met? Please consider each unit separately when answering questions 1A through 1H.

A. **Review: Is the Baby Sick?** ....

all met   half met   none met

B. **Preparation for Neonatal Transport** ....

all met   half met   none met

C. **Direct Blood Pressure Measurement** ....

all met   half met   none met

D. **Exchange, Reduction, Direct Transfusions** ....

all met   half met   none met

E. **CPAP** ....…....................

all met   half met   none met

F. **Assisted Ventilation With Mechanical Ventilators** ....

all met   half met   none met

G. **Surfactant Therapy** ....

all met   half met   none met

H. **Continuing Care for At-Risk Infants** ....

all met   half met   none met

2. How useful is the material in this book to your work?

very useful   not at all useful

3. How effectively was the material in this book conveyed?

not at all effectively   very effectively

4. How confident do you feel that you know the material in this book?

very confident   not at all confident

5. What is your overall impression of this book?

very basic   very advanced

confusing, hard to follow   clearly written, easy to follow

liked it   disliked it

Complete this form, cut it out, and submit it with your test answer sheet. It is required for *AMA PRA Category 1 Credit(s)*™ or contact hours. If you are participating in the Perinatal Continuing Education Program through a regional outreach program, a copy may also be needed by the outreach center. See the first page in this book for further information or visit www.pcep.org/cec.html.

PCEP

Perinatal Continuing Education Program

Answer Sheet
Book III: Specialized Newborn Care
Unit 1: Review: Is the Baby Sick?

Pretest

1A. Yes   No
- ___ ___ Supplemental oxygen
- ___ ___ Gestational age and size exam
- ___ ___ Blood glucose screening test
- ___ ___ Start IV, give glucose
- ___ ___ Frequent vital signs

1B. Yes   No
- ___ ___ SGA
- ___ ___ Preterm
- ___ ___ LGA
- ___ ___ Post-term

1C. Yes   No
- ___ ___ Hypoglycemia
- ___ ___ Diarrhea
- ___ ___ Meconium aspiration
- ___ ___ RDS
- ___ ___ Neonatal diabetes

1D. Yes   No
- ___ ___ Start oral feeding
- ___ ___ Antibiotics
- ___ ___ Phototherapy lights
- ___ ___ Repeat blood glucose screening test
- ___ ___ Oxygen
- ___ ___ Healthy, full term

2A. Do   Sev.   Not
     Immed.   Min.   Indicated
- ___ ___ ___ Blood glucose screening test
- ___ ___ ___ Epinephrine
- ___ ___ ___ Connect oximeter
- ___ ___ ___ Bag and mask ventilation
- ___ ___ ___ Stimulate with water
- ___ ___ ___ Hematocrit
- ___ ___ ___ Blood pressure
- ___ ___ ___ Blood gas
- ___ ___ ___ Temperature

2B. Yes   No
- ___ ___ Common problem
- ___ ___ Sepsis
- ___ ___ Hypoglycemia
- ___ ___ Aspirated formula
- ___ ___ Blood oxygen too high

Posttest

1A. Yes   No
- ___ ___ Temperature
- ___ ___ Blood pressure
- ___ ___ Hematocrit
- ___ ___ Blood glucose screening test
- ___ ___ Oxygen
- ___ ___ Oximeter

1B. Yes   No
- ___ ___ Normal saline IV bolus, slowly
- ___ ___ Normal saline IV bolus, quickly
- ___ ___ Early feeding
- ___ ___ Arterial blood gas
- ___ ___ Chest X-ray
- ___ ___ Cardiorespiratory monitor

1C. Yes   No
- ___ ___ Type and cross-match blood
- ___ ___ IV sodium bicarbonate
- ___ ___ IV glucose
- ___ ___ Bath
- ___ ___ Increase oxygen
- ___ ___ Insert UAC

1D. A   B   C   D

2A. Yes   No
- ___ ___ Chest compressions
- ___ ___ Antibiotics
- ___ ___ Restrict oxygen
- ___ ___ Ventilation

2B. Yes   No
- ___ ___ Blood pH
- ___ ___ Blood glucose screening test
- ___ ___ Bathe baby
- ___ ___ Hematocrit
- ___ ___ Blood pressure
- ___ ___ Physical and gest. age exam
- ___ ___ Temperature

2C. Yes   No
- ___ ___ Reintubate, assist ventilation
- ___ ___ IV sodium bicarbonate
- ___ ___ Chest compressions
- ___ ___ Portable x-ray
- ___ ___ Blood transfusion
- ___ ___ Glucose, slow IV push

Unit 2: Preparation for Neonatal Transport

Pretest

1A. Yes No

___ ___ Oxygen
___ ___ Send to X-ray
___ ___ Tube feeding
___ ___ Arterial blood gas
___ ___ Blood glucose test screening test
___ ___ Pulse oximeter

1B. A B C D

2. Yes No

___ ___ Peripheral IV
___ ___ Blood culture
___ ___ Blood glucose screening test
___ ___ Blood pressure
___ ___ Electrocardiogram

3. A B C D

4. Yes No

___ ___ Oxygen
___ ___ Blood glucose screening test
___ ___ Chest x-ray
___ ___ Insert UAC
___ ___ Peripheral IV
___ ___ Feed by mouth

5. Yes No

___ ___ Sodium bicarbonate
___ ___ Bag and mask
___ ___ Intubate and ventilate
___ ___ Increase oxygen

6. Yes No

___ ___ Antibiotics, then blood culture
___ ___ Insert IV
___ ___ Hematocrit
___ ___ Blood glucose screening test
___ ___ Tube feeding
___ ___ Blood gas
___ ___ Weigh baby

7. Yes No

___ ___ Blood pressure
___ ___ Repeat blood glucose screening test
___ ___ Oxygen
___ ___ Chest x-ray

8. True False

Posttest

1. A B C D
2. True False
3. Yes No

___ ___ Glucose
___ ___ Calcium
___ ___ Lumbar puncture

4. Yes No

___ ___ Crossmatch blood
___ ___ Serum calcium
___ ___ Phenobarbital
___ ___ Hematocrit

5. Yes No

___ ___ Start IV
___ ___ Give fluid
___ ___ Blood gas
___ ___ Chest x-ray
___ ___ Blood glucose screening test
___ ___ Lumbar puncture

6. Yes No

___ ___ Volume expander
___ ___ Oxygen
___ ___ Warm baby
___ ___ Hematocrit
___ ___ Chest x-ray
___ ___ Begin IV
___ ___ Feed by mouth
___ ___ Bathe baby

7. Yes No

___ ___ Skull x-ray
___ ___ Blood gas
___ ___ Oxygen
___ ___ Blood volume expander
___ ___ Breath sounds
___ ___ Chest x-ray

8A. Yes No

___ ___ Oxyhood
___ ___ Send to x-ray
___ ___ Tube feedings
___ ___ Arterial blood gas
___ ___ Blood glucose screening test

8B. A B C D

Unit 3: Direct Blood Pressure Measurement

Pretest

1. A B C D
2. True False
3. True False
4. True False
5. True False
6. A B C D
7. A B C D

Posttest

1. A B C D
2. A B C D
3. True False
4. True False
5. True False
6. A B C D
7. A B C D

Unit 4: Exchange, Reduction, and Direct Transfusions

Pretest

1. True False
2. True False
3. True False
4. True False
5. A B C D
6. A B C D
7. A B C D
8. True False
9. True False
10. True False
11. True False
12. A B C D
13. A B C D
14. A B C D

Posttest

1. True False
2. True False
3. True False
4. True False
5. A B C D
6. A B C D
7. A B C D
8. A B C D
9. A B C D
10. A B C D
11. A B C D
12. A B C D
13. True False
14. True False

Unit 5: CPAP

Pretest

1. A B C D
2. A B C D
3. True False
4. A B C D
5. A B C D
6. A B C D

Posttest

1. True False
2. True False
3. A B C D
4. A B C D
5. A B C D
6. A B C D

Unit 6: Assisted Ventilation With Mechanical Ventilators

Pretest

1. A B C D E
2. A B C D E
3. A B C D
4. A B C D
5. A B C D
6. A B C D

Posttest

1. A B C
2. A B C D
3. A B C D
4. A B C D
5. A B C D
6. A B C D

Unit 7: Surfactant Therapy

Pretest

1. A B C D
2. A B C D
3. A B C D
4. A B C D
5. A B
6. A B C D
7. True False
8. True False
9. True False
10. True False
11. True False

Posttest

1. A B C D
2. A B C D
3. A B C D
4. A B C D
5. A B C D
6. A B C D
7. True False
8. True False
9. True False
10. True False

Unit 8: Continuing Care for At-Risk Infants

Pretest

1. A B C D
2. Yes No
   ___ ___ Social Service consult
   ___ ___ Call parents
   ___ ___ Begin foster home plans
3. A B C D
4. A B C D
5. Yes No
   ___ ___ Head circumference weekly
   ___ ___ Start phenobarbital
   ___ ___ Weigh baby daily
   ___ ___ Give Imferon
   ___ ___ Hematocrit weekly
   ___ ___ Attach cardiac or respiratory monitor
6. True False
7. True False
8. True False
9. True False
10. True False
11. True False
12. True False
13. True False
14. A B C
15. A B
16. A B C D
17. Yes No
   ___ ___ Blood electrolytes
   ___ ___ Urine output
   ___ ___ Stool pH
   ___ ___ Hematocrit
   ___ ___ Weight gain
   ___ ___ Blood calcium

Posttest

1. A B C D
2. A B C D
3. A B C D
4. Yes No
   ___ ___ Assess caloric intake
   ___ ___ Assess baby's temperature
   ___ ___ Assess baby's blood pH
   ___ ___ Evaluate for infection
5. True False
6. True False
7. True False
8. True False
9. True False
10. True False
11. True False
12. True False
13. A B C D
14. A B C D
15. Yes No
   ___ ___ Stool pH
   ___ ___ Blood electrolytes
   ___ ___ Feed by NG or OG tube
   ___ ___ Incubator
   ___ ___ Administer antibiotics
16. A B C D
17. A B C D